D0780923

The **PROFESSIONAL PORTFOLIO** in **OCCUPATIONAL THERAPY**

Career Development and Continuing Competence

The PROFESSIONAL PORTFOLIO in OCCUPATIONAL THERAPY

Career Development and Continuing Competence

Janet Nagayda, OTD, MS, OTR

Saginaw Valley State University
University Center, MI

Sarah Schindehette, OTR

Chicago, IL

Jaclyn Richardson, OTR

Marlette, MI

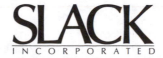

SLACK
INCORPORATED

An innovative information, education, and management company
6900 Grove Road • Thorofare, NJ 08086

ISBN-10: 1-55642-644-5
ISBN-13: 978-1-55642-644-5

Copyright © 2005 by SLACK Incorporated

All rights reserved. No part of this book may be reproduced, stored in a retrieval system or transmitted in any form or by any means, electronic, mechanical, photocopying, recording or otherwise, without written permission from the publisher, except for brief quotations embodied in critical articles and reviews.

The work SLACK Incorporated publishes is peer reviewed. Prior to publication, recognized leaders in the field, educators, and clinicians provide important feedback on the concept and content that we publish. We welcome feedback on this work.

Printed in the United States of America.

Library of Congress Cataloging-in-Publication Data
Nagayda, Janet.
    The professional portfolio in occupational therapy : career development and continuing competence / Janet Nagayda, Sarah Schindehette, Jaclyn Richardson.
      p. ; cm.
   Includes index.
   ISBN-13: 978-1-55642-644-5 (alk. paper)
   ISBN-10: 1-55642-644-5 (alk. paper)
   1. Occupational therapy. 2. Occupational therapy assistants. 3. Employment portfolios.
   [DNLM: 1. Occupational Therapy. 2. Career Mobility. 3. Professional Competence. WB 555 N147p 2005] I. Schindehette, Sarah. II. Richardson, Jaclyn. III. Title.

RM735.4.N34 2005
615.8'515--dc22

                                    2004028126

Published by: SLACK Incorporated
                 6900 Grove Road
                 Thorofare, NJ 08086 USA
                 Telephone: 856-848-1000
                 Fax: 856-853-5991
                 www.slackbooks.com

Contact SLACK Incorporated for more information about other books in this field or about the availability of our books from distributors outside the United States.

For permission to reprint material in another publication, contact SLACK Incorporated. Authorization to photocopy items for internal, personal, or academic use is granted by SLACK Incorporated provided that the appropriate fee is paid directly to Copyright Clearance Center. Prior to photocopying items, please contact the Copyright Clearance Center at 222 Rosewood Drive, Danvers, MA 01923 USA; phone: 978-750-8400; Web site: www.copyright.com; email: info@copyright.com

Last digit is print number: 10   9   8   7   6   5   4   3   2   1

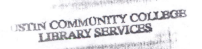
AUSTIN COMMUNITY COLLEGE
LIBRARY SERVICES

DEDICATION

We dedicate this book to family, friends, and colleagues for their unending support and patience during the inception and fulfillment of this project.

CONTENTS

ACKNOWLEDGMENTS

We would like to acknowledge the faculty, students, and alumni of the Occupational Therapy Program at Saginaw Valley State University for the feedback and inspiration we received as they have engaged in the portfolio creation process over the last twelve years. Their efforts and outcomes inspired us to formalize the process for the benefit of others.

ABOUT THE AUTHORS

Janet Nagayda, OTD, MS, OTR, is the acting Program Director of the Occupational Therapy Program at Saginaw Valley State University in Michigan. She has been an occupational therapist for over thirty years and in academia for thirteen years. Her primary practice areas have been school-based service, the application of assistive technology, and program and curriculum development.

Sarah Schindehette, OTR, has been an occupational therapist with the adult population in a variety of service settings. She is currently applying her skills in the business world as a regional Vice President of a financial services organization. Her long-term professional goals include owning and managing a private rehabilitation enterprise and teaching.

Jaclyn Richardson, OTR, is currently in part-time practice in an inpatient rehabilitation setting. A toddler and new baby are receiving her primary attention. Jackie has also worked closely with a home building group to develop adaptive living spaces.

PREFACE

A primary concern for the profession of occupational therapy has been the promotion of public awareness and demand for occupational therapy services. Integral to achievement of these ends is the need for occupational therapy practitioners to define and plan their own career path and effectively articulate their capabilities to those outside the profession. The National Board for Certification in Occupational Therapy has recently underscored the need for professional planning and continuing education with implementation of revised certification standards. The use of a portfolio system can help occupational therapy practitioners plan, execute, and verify participation in activities to meet all these objectives as well as to promote the individual and the profession through a clear and organized presentation of professional and personal activities spanning the career. This book assists the reader in defining personal objectives and identifies a pathway toward portfolio development.

Foundations

Occupational Therapy Defined

Definition of Occupational Therapy

"…the art and science of directing man's participation in selected tasks to restore, reinforce, and enhance performance; facilitate learning of those skills and functions that are essential for adaptation and productivity; diminish or correct pathology; and promote and maintain health. Its fundamental concern is the development and maintenance of capacity throughout the life span, to perform with satisfaction to self and others, those tasks and roles essential to productive living and to the mastery of self and environment" (American Occupational Therapy Association, 1972).

WHAT IS OCCUPATIONAL THERAPY?

Who are occupational therapists and what do they do? Whether you are an occupational therapy student or an occupational therapy practitioner, you have likely been asked this question countless times. How you respond is a reflection of how you feel about the profession and your role in it.

The definition of occupational therapy has many uses. It forms a foundation for the philosophical base, provides parameters for practice processes, and gives some guidance to the practitioner for professional growth. The definition may not be as useful to others outside of the profession. It may not facilitate a clear visualization of how occupational therapy fits within their organization or could be of benefit with a particular population. Occupational therapy practitioners may find it helpful, or even necessary, to have a clear, more graphic representation of the profession and personal experiences.

Occupational therapy practitioners are goal-oriented individuals who assess client needs, skills, and abilities within related contexts, and then help develop goals and plans to achieve them. The goals of treatment may be as diverse as the population occupational therapists serve. They should, however, have one common theme: increasing independence and function. Occupational therapy practitioners assist people of all ages and from all backgrounds to more fully engage their life roles in meaningful ways.

PROFESSIONAL ROLES

There are two levels of occupational therapy practice. The registered occupational therapist (OTR) is educated to the bachelor or master's degree level and is certified for entry-level practice. At the level of client service, the OTR is able to evaluate and intervene with individuals evidencing a myriad of impairments, disabilities, and/or handicaps. He or she assesses, collects, and interprets data; identifies underlying problems affecting individual performance; and develops an intervention plan suited to the needs of a particular client. An occupational therapy assistant (OTA) is a certified professional with an associate degree level of education. The OTA collaborates with the OTR to develop and implement treat-

Personal Application Guide

Reflective Thinking

➤ What does being an occupational therapist or occupational therapy assistant mean to you?

_____

_____

_____

➤ How have you used the skills you have developed in your professional role in other aspects of your life?

_____

_____

_____

➤ How has being an occupational therapy practitioner enhanced your ability to cope, plan, organize, and facilitate activities outside the scope of your practice?

_____

_____

_____

➤ How, in developing a professional portfolio, can you help others to not only understand what occupational therapy is, but how you can direct your expertise in new and exciting directions? Who could benefit from this education?

_____

_____

_____

ment plans that will promote independence and increase functional ability for clients (Bureau of Labor Statistics, 2002-2003). The OTR and OTA expanded roles also typically encompass administrative, supervisory, educational, program develop-ment, entrepreneurial, public relations, research, and countless other activities. Many of these functions are not blatantly obvious but are no less important and require the development of relevant specialized skills.

Personal Application Guide

Reflective Thinking: Sample Response

➤ What does being an occupational therapist or occupational therapy assistant mean to you?

As an occupational therapist, I am able to help people regain a level of functioning and independence that they would not be able to achieve otherwise. I am able to help people regain their freedom, self-worth, and dignity by using skills that I have learned throughout my training process and my experiences with a variety of patients. I am honored to be in a profession where I not only teach my patients skills, but more importantly, they teach me about living.

➤ How have you used the skills you have developed in your professional role in other aspects of your life?

I have learned patience, motivational skills, effective interpersonal communication, time management, greater empathy for others, and a thirst for continuing self-improvement. All these skills help me in my everyday life from raising my children to teaching Sunday School.

➤ How has being an occupational therapy practitioner enhanced your ability to cope, plan, organize, and facilitate activities outside the scope of your practice?

Every day, I teach people how to effectively cope with their situation and improve upon it, compose a successful treatment plan to reach their goals, and facilitate activities to improve their level of functioning. Because I am constantly teaching these skills, I internalize them. Often without realizing it, I find that I am using these same skills to handle my daily stresses by working to find better ways of organizing my time and facilitating independence in those close to me so that they can shoulder some of the stresses.

➤ How, in developing a professional portfolio, can you help others to not only understand what occupational therapy is, but how you can direct your expertise in new and exciting directions? Who could benefit from this education?

By having a professional portfolio, I would be able to give people a visual overview of what I do, so that they would have a clear mental picture instead of me giving a brief verbal description that they may not understand or that they will quickly forget. Many of the doctors that I work with would benefit from seeing all of the areas in which I can effectively help patients.

Portfolios and Pitch Books

PORTFOLIOS AND PITCH BOOKS DEFINED

The portfolio format has long been used as a means to identify skills that are integral to a particular profession and to provide a visual representation of an individual's knowledge and expertise. The artist, architect, interior designer, and others use the portfolio as a means to showcase their talents. Teachers develop and maintain portfolios to demonstrate their skills and experiences in academic settings. As an occupational therapist or occupational therapy assistant, you can also benefit from using this format to document your achievements and plan professional growth.

A portfolio system is a method of information management aimed at helping all occupational therapy professionals showcase and direct their professional experiences and development (the specifics of this system are discussed in Section 2). From this point forward, the term *occupational therapy practitioner* will refer to both the occupational therapist and the occupational therapy assistant. The respective title will be used if it becomes necessary to make a distinction. This guide to professional development through the creation of a professional portfolio system is relevant to all occupational therapy practitioners at both levels of practice and all levels of experience, wherever your career takes you.

A portfolio is a visual representation of personal and professional goals and accomplishments. It has been said that goals that aren't written are merely wishes. Every stage of the portfolio development process necessitates goal setting, periodic review, and then the appropriate adjustments. The familiar format of the occupational therapy process could be invoked to facilitate your thinking and preparations.

* Screening/referral: What is the purpose of the portfolio for you?

* Assessment: How have your past experiences prepared you for your current endeavor? What are the related strengths and weaknesses?

* Goals: What do you want to accomplish now and in the future?

* Intervention plan: What do you need to do to prepare yourself? This may include formal or continuing education, a mentor, volunteer experience, reflective thought, or any other experience that will move you closer to your goals.

* Reassessment: This review will help you decide whether or not you have met your goals successfully.

A *portfolio* helps professionals define and track professional and personal goals. First, you look at what you want your portfolio to say about you, the result you want to see, and how you might go about achieving it. After the portfolio is completed, you will periodically review it to see if it needs to be updated. One of the purposes of the portfolio is to establish a tracking system to maintain an accurate record of expanding skills, interests, and continuing education. You will then customize the portfolio to meet your own unique needs and style.

A *pitch book* is a streamlined version of your portfolio that can be used to provide a highly focused look at your skills and abilities or those of your business, private practice, or special project. You will be able to quickly and effectively give your audience a lasting visual of the positive impact that you, your business, or special event can bring them. Not only will it spark their interest, but also will give them enough evidence to confidently select you.

Why Create Portfolios and Pitch Books?

The portfolio and pitch book demonstrate your continued individual professionalism and the professional status of the field as a whole. Professional beliefs and values shape the choices you make and the actions you take. During the academic years, students are socialized into their chosen profession. Underlying values are developed and guide growth within the profession (Abbott, 1988). The identification and expression of these beliefs infuses your professional relationships and helps you identify yourself as a member of a larger group—occupational therapy.

Sullivan (1995) defines a professional as having several specific characteristics:

* Specialized training in a field of defined knowledge
* Public recognition of a community of practitioners to regulate standards of practice
* A commitment to provide service to the public beyond the practitioner's own economic welfare
* The acquisition of professional credentials

This definition requires that practitioners meet very special requirements and acquire necessary skills. It further requires providing the best service to all those in need regardless of any economic gain or lack thereof. The parameters of occupational therapy have been delineated in the *Uniform Terminology for Occupational Therapy 3rd Edition* (American Occupational Therapy Association, 1994) and in the more recent *Occupational Therapy Practice Framework: Domain and Process* (AOTA, 2002). Standards of practice have been made available by the AOTA to guide intervention across the field and are continually being revised to reflect best practice. State and national practice boards, such as the National Board for Certification of Occupational Therapy (NBCOT), and educational accrediting agencies, such as the American Council for Occupational Therapy Education (ACOTE), are charged with monitoring professional practice. *The Occupational Therapy Code*

of Ethics (AOTA, 1994) provides standards for the ethical management of professional affairs and inter- actions with clients and families, coworkers, and all others involved in the day-to-day activities of occupational therapy practitioners' professional lives. Every occupational therapist approved to practice must demonstrate the acquisition and performance of a set of defined skills at a specified level of competency and behavior. There is an agreed upon code of behavior and a continuum of skills to guide and facilitate the enactment of your professional services as an occupational therapist.

Professional integrity requires the practitioner to make a commitment to caring, learning, and applying ethical and effective treatment. To do this, you must have considerable self-awareness and commitment (Sullivan, 1995). The systematic development of a portfolio system facilitates the self-examination required of the professional person and by maintaining the system you can ensure that growth continues. A portfolio should then reflect your membership within a particular profession, the internalization of its core values, and the attainment of an agreed upon level of skill, as well as evidence that you plan to continue growing and learning within professional guidelines.

Portfolios and pitch books are valuable to both the individual practitioner and the profession as a whole. When occupational therapy practitioners use a portfolio system, it provides an excellent educational opportunity for the community at large. Whenever portfolios are presented, especially to those outside the profession, it affords an opportunity for consumers, reimbursement agents, service agencies, and others to be treated to a small presentation on what occupational therapy is and what its practitioners can do. This is hugely important as you move into new service areas and work toward expanding existing ones.

The portfolio system and the process of completing, reviewing, and updating your portfolio and pitch book, as well as the completed product, can be beneficial for every occupational therapy professional, in every setting, and at every stage in the career. Some of the foundational benefits are evaluation, including certification and accreditation processes; professional development; and employment.

Evaluation

There are several types of evaluation in which you may engage. One is a process of self-examination. The individual takes an honest look at personal and/or professional growth, skills, talents, and expe-

Student Testimonial

In the OT program at my university, it was required to have a professional portfolio completed prior to graduation. Throughout the two years of the program, I collected and compiled documents that I felt would help to represent me as a skilled and valuable clinician. From a student's perspective, it was a great tool to help develop myself as a professional.

I found that the portfolio has been helpful to use for interviews, business proposals, job promotions, and a resource for recertification requirements. It serves as an excellent resource to show others what I have accomplished, what I continue to work on, and what future plans I may have. It can also provide personal satisfaction when I can walk away from a situation and know that there is not one thing that I forgot to say because I had it all right there in front of me. Overall, I look at the portfolio as my future and a way for me, as well as others, to see my professional growth.

Jean Krueger

riences; determines strengths and weaknesses; and identifies needs. There are also certification/regulation evaluations like those required by state and national professional boards for approval to practice. Requirements may include standardized testing, continuing education, and other professional activities as a requirement. Another type of evaluation process may occur in the work place where specific criteria must be met for continuing employment, promotion, or special recognition, such as merit raises or awards. This is particularly helpful when the evaluator is unfamiliar with the scope of occupational therapy. With the changing health care environment, it is becoming more crucial to be able to demonstrate initial and continued competence to your employers, regulatory boards, clients and other constituents, and the public. The portfolio system can be used as a planning, tracking, and exhibition medium to facilitate the record keeping inherent in all of these types of evaluation.

Professional Development

In this instance, the portfolio serves as a means of planning and tracking continuing education and other professional development activities. It gives you the chance to take stock of the choices you have made and perhaps make some necessary changes. There are so many choices available to increase your knowledge and skills and engage in personal development activities, that without a cohesive and comprehensive plan, you could easily spend a great deal of time and money without getting the desired result.

Employment

The portfolio and pitch book are invaluable during the job-seeking and interviewing processes. As you consider your next employment adventure, the contents of the portfolio can help you focus on the practice areas for which you are most qualified and illuminate existing and developing areas of interest. It will help you determine bodies of knowledge and skills that require additional study or training as you prepare for a desired move.

Once you have decided on a direction, the portfolio can help you prepare for the interview process. Research of the organization, its mission, and details of the desired position will allow you to structure the portfolio and pitch book to highlight your abilities as they relate to these expectations. At the interview, you can use the portfolio to provide visual support for the questions asked and generate questions more closely aligned with your own experiences and strengths. It will be readily apparent why you are the best choice for the job at hand.

Student

You can benefit from the development and use of a portfolio system at any point in your professional life. During your academic years, you will find that developing a portfolio of accomplishments underscores the value of class work and fieldwork learning activities. As a student, you are better able to take a holistic view of these activities to see how each fits into the larger picture of practice. It leads you to more fully embrace the curriculum and motivates you to take advantage of a broader range of opportunities and experiences that might not previously

Entry-Level Practitioner Testimonial

Completing a professional portfolio has had a tremendously positive impact on my professional life and development. The professional portfolio has consistently impressed interviewers, and I believe it has helped me earn employment opportunities. I brought my portfolio to every professional interview in which I have participated. In every instance the interviewer has spent significant time browsing the portfolio, and in every instance the interviewer has given me positive verbal feedback. One interviewer actually read aloud a line from a past performance review regarding timeliness of documentation, and shook her head enthusiastically in positive acknowledgement. I must add that this particular interviewer revealed to me several months after I had accepted a position that the portfolio highly impressed her, and had clinched her decision to offer me the position. I strongly believe that looking at tangible photographs, award certificates, performance evaluations, work samples, and the like has an intensely powerful impact on an interviewer; exponentially more powerful than the words of the interviewee alone.

The portfolio also provides a document that brings together the sum of my accomplishments. The act of looking back at the portfolio prior to an interview has provided me with an opportunity to internally organize my past achievements, so I have been completely prepared to answer any question about my educational, professional, and community service background.

In summary, the professional portfolio has provided me with an organized, personal, and thorough summary of my accomplishments in an interesting format. I honestly believe that the portfolio has given me a distinct advantage in the achievement of a rewarding professional career. I would recommend constructing and maintaining a portfolio to any prospective health care professional!

David Weiss

have been considered. It also provides a good organizational tool to integrate what you have learned as you prepare for the national registration examination.

Entry-Level

As an entry-level practitioner, you will need to gain confidence in your ability as an occupational therapy practitioner. Your academic program began the professional socialization process and the first year or two of employment will continue the process. The act of putting together a portfolio system will help you reflect on the whole of your education and clinical experiences. In the beginning, it is only natural to be unsure of your abilities and it is very reassuring to actually see what you have accomplished. It can really prepare the entry-level practitioner for those first job interviews.

Intermediate

The intermediate level practitioner is most likely focused on refining personal and professional strengths and interests. This is also a time when you will assess your selection of a career path and make important decisions regarding higher education. The portfolio system assists you by providing an organized look at what you have accomplished and highlights areas of interest and particular skills. It also

requires that you identify and acknowledge those skill areas that are not as strong. Where should you focus your continuing education efforts to receive the most return in terms of personal growth, time, and money? Is it time to seek that promotion or perhaps new employment? These are weighty issues requiring a clear, unflinching look at your needs and strengths, accomplishments, and desires for the future.

Advanced

Advanced career practitioners may find that they are ready for a change, either into a new area on their existing career path or something totally different. When you reach this point in your career, the portfolio may help clarify possible options by revealing areas of interest and highlighting strengths. It will help you validate your experiences and skills as you move into new waters.

Re-Entry

The re-entry practitioner will find a portfolio system helpful whether he or she is developing a new portfolio or updating an existing one. The process will highlight strengths and any areas of concern. The portfolio allows you to incorporate skills in all areas, including the time you may have been away from practice. It also assists you in determining what

Intermediate Practitioner Testimonial

In college, I had some really great experiences in my fieldwork and externships. I got to see and experience many facets of occupational therapy from outpatient therapy and pediatrics to mental health and home care. Coming out of the occupational therapy program in 1995, a portfolio wasn't a requirement of graduation. Back then, occupational therapy jobs were in high demand and a dime a dozen. I put everything I could into a resume, but it is difficult to sum up all of my experiences and accomplishments into one or two pages. I got the first job I applied for, which was in sub-acute care rehab.

Since then, I have decided sub-acute care isn't my forte and went out in search of a new job. I had my resume in hand, but nothing to show or prove my experience. The job I applied for was in outpatient therapy with occasional inpatient and home care rehab. I got the job, but several times I felt that there was so much more I could do as an outpatient therapist, but didn't have the resources readily available to market myself to administration. Also, if I wanted to relocate and/or change jobs completely and get out of the outpatient area of occupational therapy practice, I could use that portfolio to draw on those past experiences and accomplishments to market myself.

Kristie Fox-Warren

Advanced Practitioner Testimonial

I had been in practice for over 15 years, 13 of those as Director of Occupational Therapy in a rural intermediate school district. I loved the work but really felt the need for a change. I had been doing too much of the same thing, with the same clientele, for too long. Moving was out of the question and the ISD was a great employer. An opportunity arose within the ISD to take a fresh look at how early intervention services were being provided to the children and their families in our county. The current director's position was being eliminated and all ideas were welcome. The administration had always felt that a speech and language pathologist presented the most appropriate qualifications for leadership of this program, but they were willing to look at all ideas. I reviewed all my past education and experiences and put together a package of ideas to present to the administration and early intervention team. No small feat! I hadn't saved much from conferences I had attended, beyond the information I had directly applied in practice. I knew I did a report on a related topic during my Master's level courses but where was it? Where were the letters parents and others had written regarding my abilities and the special activities I had been involved in? I managed to pull together a nice presentation, but it was difficult and more time consuming than it needed to be.

Janet Nagayda

needs to be done to prepare for a return to the work force. Do you need to update specific skills? Would volunteer work be helpful? What continuing education is needed? The portfolio will help build confidence in your ability to return to work because you will be able to be objective in developing a plan for your return.

Indirect or Nontraditional

The portfolio system will be especially helpful for you at any point in your career when working in indirect or nontraditional roles. It will help to demonstrate how what you know as an occupational therapy practitioner can be translated into the successful performance of a wide variety of jobs that aren't thought of specifically as occupational therapy.

Your professional values, viewpoints, knowledge base, and personal skills are apparent in a well-developed portfolio system and will support your move into other areas of service.

CONCLUSION

Creating a portfolio system facilitates your ability to see yourself in what is perhaps a new way by shining a light on your current skills, abilities, and interests while helping you define your true professional goals. Dreams may evolve that you hadn't even considered, or perhaps you will rediscover some you had forgotten about! You can use this system to assist you in determining where you are now, where you

Re-Entry Practitioner Testimonial

I am currently not working in the occupational therapy field. In fact, I am working in the financial arena, where I educate families on how to get out of debt and become financially independent. In addition to working with families, I am also in charge of hiring, training, and developing people in management and leadership positions for several office locations. While this may seem drastically different from occupational therapy, it's similar because I use the same skills in both settings: educating, training, motivating, evaluating, and devising an appropriate plan of action, etc. My training as a therapist has prepared me for my current endeavors. I love what I am doing now, but my long-term goal is to open up a pediatric rehabilitation center with a nonprofit component. My current position is affording me an opportunity to develop a new set of skills in business and finances, which I will need when opening up my own center. I use my portfolio to help me plan and track my career path so that I stay current in both areas. I am maintaining my licenses, attending conferences, and presenting and publishing in occupational therapy, all in preparation for opening my pediatric business in the future. Because I created and am maintaining my portfolio, I will be prepared to show how all of my time and experience in the business world, in addition to my continuing efforts in occupational therapy, translate into competence to open and run a pediatric facility.

Sarah Schindehette

Indirect or Nontraditional Practitioner Testimonial

I had been thinking for several years that I would like to move my career into the academic realm. I had never taught—what in the world made me think I could do this? I began to look at my teaching skills. I came to realize that occupational therapists ARE teachers. We take on a teaching role with our clients, their families, the service team, a wide variety of community members—anyone who'll stand still long enough to listen. What about writing? I write constantly in my practice with client evaluations, program planning and implementation, progress notes, and so on. I had also taken a small plunge into writing for publication. Research? I hadn't done any beyond my clinical-based efforts, but I realized that program planning, implementation, data collection, and reviewing the results was the basis for developing research skills. What did I need to do to further prepare myself? I had a Master's of Science degree in Occupational Therapy Administration and was looking into doctoral study options. I accepted an evening adjunct teaching position to try out the classroom. I taught medical terminology to get my feet wet and then tackled anatomy physiology. I loved it and began looking for a full-time position. It was time for a big change. A portfolio would have made this discovery process easier, and perhaps I would have come to it sooner. I could have prepared in a more organized way and taken better advantages of opportunities.

Janet Nagayda

want to go, and exactly how you are going to get there. Think about this: when you go on an extended road trip you probably spend a lot of time planning not only where you want to travel and stay, but also how to get there and what you want to do when you arrive. So, why wouldn't you do the same for your career? The cathartic process of designing your portfolio helps you to make wonderful discoveries about who you are, what destination you want to reach, and if you are on the right track to get there. If you find that you are not on the path you want, then the portfolio system will help you to plan a more satisfying journey.

Personal Application Guide

Choosing a Career Path

Occupational therapy offers an enormous array of opportunities and settings in which to practice. The chart below demonstrates a fraction of these options. Next to each setting that applies, write a brief description of your experience (when, how long, level of expertise in this area, etc.). Then, place a star next to any settings that you would like to gain some skill in now or in the future. At the bottom of the page, list and describe any areas not mentioned that you have experience in or would like to explore further.

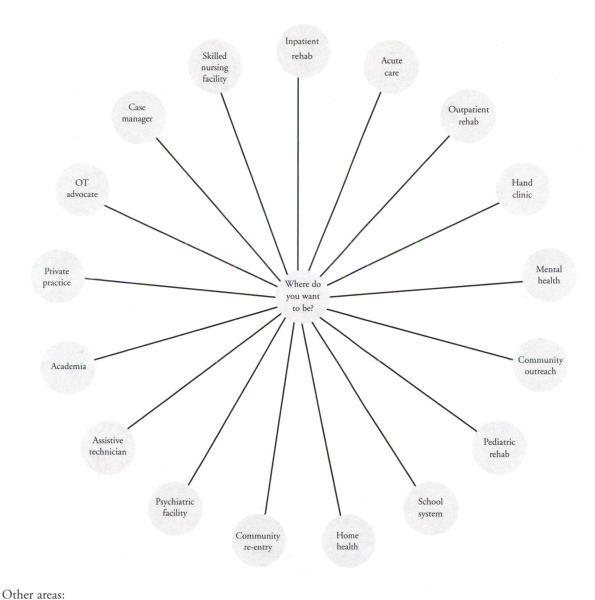

Other areas:

_____

_____

_____

Personal Application Guide

Choosing a Career Path: Sample Response

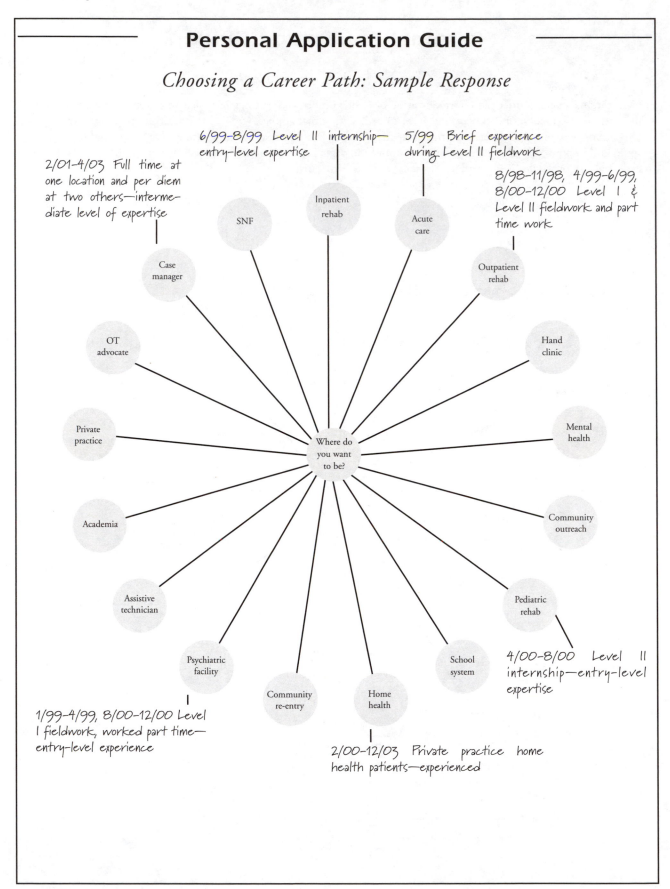

6/99–8/99 Level II internship—entry-level expertise

5/99 Brief experience during Level II fieldwork

2/01–4/03 Full time at one location and per diem at two others—intermediate level of expertise

8/98–11/98, 4/99–6/99, 8/00–12/00 Level I & Level II fieldwork and part time work

SNF

Inpatient rehab

Acute care

Case manager

Outpatient rehab

OT advocate

Hand clinic

Private practice

Mental health

Where do you want to be?

Academia

Community outreach

Assistive technician

Pediatric rehab

Psychiatric facility

Community re-entry

Home health

School system

4/00–8/00 Level II internship—entry-level expertise

1/99–4/99, 8/00–12/00 Level I fieldwork, worked part time—entry-level experience

2/00–12/03 Private practice home health patients—experienced

Personal Application Guide

Choosing a Career Path

Just like there are countless settings in which to practice, there are also countless career paths to take. These paths can be horizontal, like in example A (from one setting or facility to another), or vertical, like in example B (gain of experience, responsibility and/or level of promotion). The combination of these two paths creates an individualized career path, like in example C.

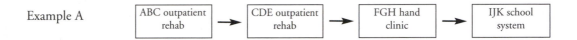

Example A   ABC outpatient rehab → CDE outpatient rehab → FGH hand clinic → IJK school system

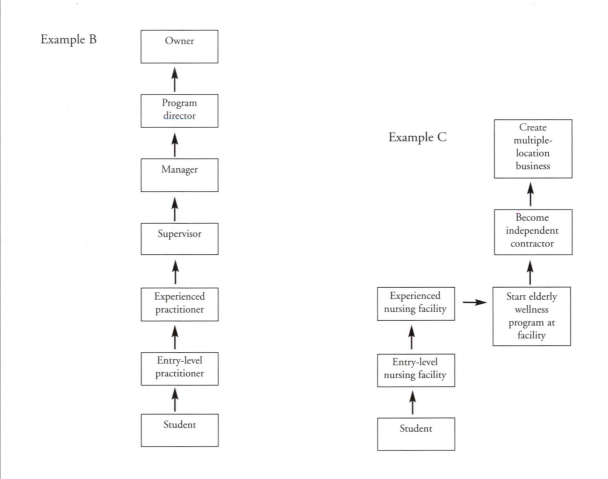

Example B

Owner
↑
Program director
↑
Manager
↑
Supervisor
↑
Experienced practitioner
↑
Entry-level practitioner
↑
Student

Example C

Create multiple-location business
↑
Become independent contractor
↑
Experienced nursing facility → Start elderly wellness program at facility
↑
Entry-level nursing facility
↑
Student

Personal Application Guide

Choosing a Career Path

What does your career path currently look like? Sketch it out.

Describe in detail what your ideal job would look like. Think about setting, position, coworkers and peers, location, the facility, income, clientele, hours, self-employment versus working for someone else, managing a staff or being managed by a supervisor, etc.

_____

_____

_____

_____

What would you like your career path to look like over the next year, five years, and 10 years? Does this path get you to your ideal job? Sketch it out.

What actions do you need to take to get on the career path that you want? Do you need more information, education, certifications, and/or experience through work or volunteering? Is there a financial aspect that needs to be planned? Who can you talk with to help you plan your next move? What could prevent you from achieving this goal? How can you overcome these obstacles?

_____

_____

_____

_____

The System and the Process

The Portfolio System

3

WHAT TO INCLUDE

The portfolio system consists of your file cabinet, portfolio, and a pitch book. The file cabinet or any other means of holding all those artifacts you don't want to part with is the genesis of your portfolio system. In it, you put all of those items you kept from school and those that accumulate from workshops and other professional experiences. During your school years, you explore many facets of occupational therapy and hear the results of work done by your peers. You are given a multitude of resources and information and have varied experiences on your fieldwork that will prove useful in the years to come. You just don't know which ones you'll need and when. Conferences, workshops, and inservices also provide you with information and skills that you are not always able to apply immediately. What do you do with the notes you took and the handouts you received? Will you be able to find them when you need them? The file cabinet system allows you to categorize and store the information and contacts for possible future use.

You should also include those items collected from personal life experiences in which you have become knowledgeable, been given recognition, or learned a skill that may be applicable in your professional development. Were you the Lions Club president, a school board member, the sailing team captain, or a scout leader? These kinds of activities provide you with leadership and team building experience, project organization and development skills, and invaluable opportunities to develop interpersonal skills. Have you served as the treasurer for your church, participated in a fund drive for Special Olympics, or put together a Bowl-a-Thon to raise money for Big Brothers/Big Sisters? You have developed important skills related to budget development and locating and obtaining funding sources. Have you spent time as a mentor for teens, tutored in reading programs for young children, or helped plan a social event for local seniors? Then you have experience with the concerns of individuals across the lifespan and empathy for their needs. Do you fly a plane, swim, sew, or have other special talents? Your career may take you in some exciting and unexpected directions and these experiences will be valuable resources for you. People with "pack rat" tendencies love this aspect of the system, but it may be a bit overwhelming for others. Providing yourself with a dedicated filing cabinet system will help you organize and safely store all of these materials so that you are able to make use of them when you need to. Organize your files in whatever way makes the most sense to you: alphabetically by title or subject, chronologically by date, or by any other useful means.

WHICH COMES FIRST?

Which comes first, the portfolio or the pitch book? The process is really the same. The finished product, however, is different. The deciding factor is your purpose. The portfolio is a varied showcase of your talents, abilities, and experience. It has more depth and breadth because it is designed to be used in many situations with varied audiences. The pitch book is a specific demonstration of what you and/or

---

Personal Application Guide

Choosing

The outpatient rehabilitation program where you are employed would like to start a new back-to-work program and will hire the new director from within the existing department. You have had an interest in this type of program for some time and have aimed your professional development toward this type of client. How can you most effectively present yourself as the best choice for the director position?

_____

_____

_____

_____

_____

_____

_____

_____

---

your business can provide, tailored for a specific audience. It is compact, with precise information and artifacts chosen expressly to elicit a desire on the part of the viewer to work with you. The portfolio is an overview of your abilities and experiences, while the pitch book is a laser-focused product allowing you to demonstrate how only you can meet an identified need.

While you don't need to have one to have the other, the objectives are so different that it is often helpful to have both the portfolio and the pitch book. Even though the pitch book would seem easiest to do first, because it is smaller and more direct, it is usually easier to create after your portfolio. You can take ideas, artifacts, and even entire pages out of your portfolio as you need them to create the desired effect for the pitch book. Completing the portfolio first allows you to perfect your process so that your pitch book flows more easily. By completing the portfolio first, you will also have a good handle on your personal skill sets, which is necessary for you to decide the most effective pieces to include in your pitch book. You must thoroughly understand something to really sell it and, in this case, you are selling yourself and occupational therapy.

PORTFOLIO OR PITCH BOOK?

The portfolio focuses on you as a whole. It will include:

* All your educational experiences
* All your experiences with program development
* An overview of all your assessment and intervention expertise
* Your overall professional development plan

The pitch book focus begins and ends with portraying you in the best possible light toward a very specific end, for example, if you wanted to start a back-to-work program. It will include:

* The educational experiences directly related to work programs
* Emphasize how your past program development experience will translate to your ability to put together an effective return-to-work program
* The assessment and intervention procedures you are proficient with related to work programs
* Your professional development plan as it pertains to supporting your skills in a return-to-work program

The Portfolio Process 4

STAGES OF THE PROCESS

The portfolio creation process consists of four stages: collecting, selecting, organizing, and displaying the information and artifacts that best meet the goals you have set. The biggest hurdle between you and the completion of your portfolio is usually just getting started. The job may seem overwhelming without a production plan. Decide when you would like to have the project completed and plan backwards to make appointments with yourself to work on the process. Don't wait until you have an interview or a job evaluation scheduled to begin. You will want to have time to find or send for the artifacts you need and give careful consideration to what is included and how best to present the information. You want to show your best effort, not just what you can throw together under pressure.

Examples of What to Collect

* Quotes that reflect your values/beliefs
* Transcripts
* Scholarship awards
* Diplomas
* Conference brochures
* Pictures of you presenting
* Samples of your documentation
* Thank-you letters and notes

Collecting

The collecting phase is probably the simplest in that you simply save anything that may be useful now or in the future. You don't need to screen items too closely at this point, but it may be helpful to at least file them within like categories. Some items may be both date and topic sensitive and could be placed in more than one category. If something can be placed in multiple categories, make a note of the item and place this note in the additional categories. In general, there are nine basic categories recommended for the beginner:

1. Values, mission, goals
2. Education
3. Professional development
4. Professional skills
5. Professional presentations
6. Professional publications
7. Service
8. Expressions of support
9. Personal

Your file cabinet or other filing device will keep items in good shape and help you find what you need, when you need it, to meet a particular purpose. Artifacts such as pictures, computer discs, and audio and video tapes will require special care for safe preservation. It is important that as you collect these items you obtain permission from individuals in your pictures and tapes in writing and/or eliminate any confidential or identifying information. Remember to comply with all copyright laws just as you would for any other document.

Personal Application Guide

Selecting the Best Artifacts

Rank the following artifacts on a scale from 1 to 5 (1 meaning you wouldn't use it, 5 being the best). Write a brief explanation as to why you ranked each one as you did and what attained skills, traits, or level of experience was inferred by each.

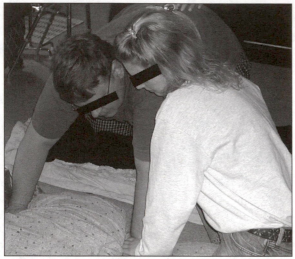

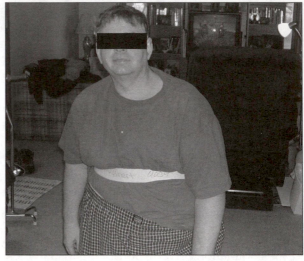

1. _____

_____

_____

_____

2. _____

_____

_____

_____

Selecting

Selecting appropriate items for use in the portfolio will depend on several things. What is your objective? Who is your audience? What is important for them to know about you? The results must be clear and concise. You will likely choose too many items in the beginning, which is to be expected. You will continually revise your choices as the development process continues. Do not throw anything away! If you do not choose to include an item in this draft, you may wish to use it at another time. Select items that demonstrate several characteristics and/or traits at once to maximize the effect and remember that you will be revising and updating your portfolio over time. Ultimately, you will maintain a loosely organized file of collected material in addition to your portfolio. This will make the selecting process easier in successive revisions to meet changing needs. The occupational therapy practitioner is qualified to work in a wide variety of settings and may be interviewing in several of these simultaneously. You may wish to select and emphasize different skills and experiences depending on the opportunities available. The focus of your portfolio can be altered to meet these varied needs.

Personal Application Guide

Selecting the Best Artifacts

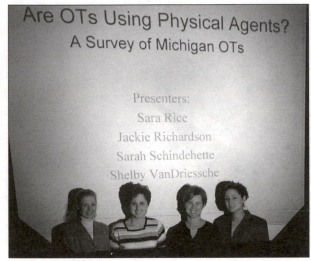

3. _____
   _____
   _____
   _____

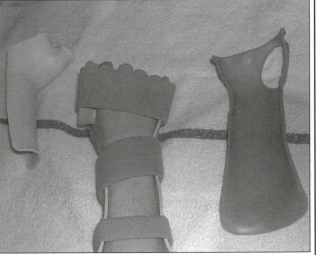

4. _____
   _____
   _____
   _____

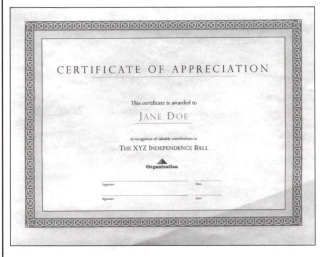

5. _____
   _____
   _____
   _____

6. _____
   _____
   _____
   _____

Personal Application Guide

Selecting the Best Artifacts

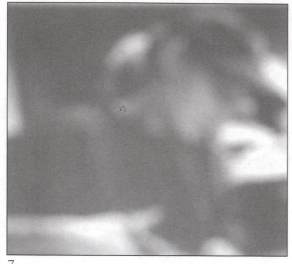

7. _____
   _____
   _____
   _____

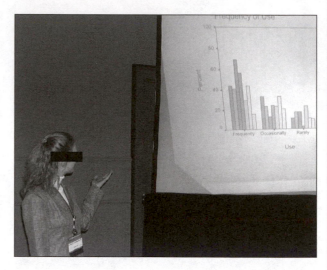

8. _____
   _____
   _____
   _____

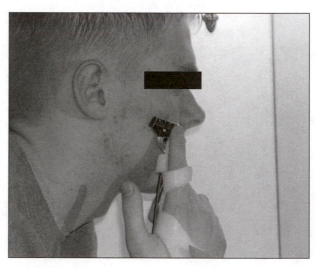

PNF

When to Use PNF

o   PNF can be used in countless ways and with a wide variety of diagnoses.

o   The emphasis of PNF is on remediating neurological deficits such as Cerebral Vascular Accident (CVA), Multiple Sclerosis (MS), Cerebral Palsy (CP), Traumatic Brain Injury (TBI), Spinal Cord Injury (SCI), Muscular Dystrophy (MD), and Parkinson's disease.

o   Some additional diagnoses that PNF is useful for include: Arthritis, Orthopedic Conditions, and Peripheral Nerve Injury.

9. _____
   _____
   _____
   _____

10. _____
    _____
    _____
    _____

Personal Application Guide

Selecting the Best Artifacts: Sample Responses

1. This is a good action photo that demonstrates NDT techniques in use, client/therapist interaction, ability to co-treat with other therapists, and home health care setting experience. I'd **rate it a 5.**

2. This is a nice picture, but it doesn't show anything; perhaps it can be used in a before-and-after shot to demonstrate progress. It would be better to show the therapist with the client. I'd **rate it a 3.**

3. I like that you can clearly read the title of the presentation, but it is difficult to see the faces of the presenters and the background is dark. I'd like to see some action demonstrated. I'd **rate it a 3.**

4. The picture shows three types of fabricated splints made out of different materials. This shows skill in developing a variety of splints for different needs. The middle splint is modeled, showing the fit and function that is required in an effective splint. I'd **rate it a 4.**

5. Certificates of appreciation are good because they lend some authenticity to many activities. It would be better to show an action photo accompanying the certificate, and a brief description of the event to add more impact. I'd **rate it 4.**

6. Brochures can be a great visual for seminars, workshops, and conferences attended. If it was a major seminar, I would show some pictures and/or a brief description of the skills learned and knowledge gained. I'd **rate it a 4.**

7. Even though this appears to be a good action photo of splint fabrication, the blurriness of the photo is disconcerting to view. I'd **rate it a 1.**

8. This is a good action photo that demonstrates experience giving professional presentations. I'd **rate it a 5.**

9. These notes don't give a good visual of what was learned or how it was applied. I'd **rate it a 1.**

10. This is a good, clear action photo. Demonstrating the adaptive shaver being used instead of just showing the shaver is much more effective. I'd **rate it a 5.**

Organizing

The way you choose to assemble your portfolio or pitch book reflects your understanding of the profession and your potential role within the profession. It is also a reflection of your personal style. Spend some time thinking about how you will use the portfolio. Chances are, the new graduate will be using nearly all of the collected material. You want to show potential employers and others that you are well rounded, have an appropriate understanding of occupational therapy, and possess the necessary professional skills. You may also find that there are some significant gaps in experience that need to be filled to meet the goals you have set. Starting this process early allows you time to increase your skill level and/or broaden your experience. If you are an experienced practitioner, consider the skills you have in your current setting that will carry over to other areas and organize the material so that this information stands out. No matter what your reason for developing the portfolio, organize it so that it makes sense to you. You should be confident with the layout and comfortable enough with the organization so that you feel a flow of information and can explain it in a logical manner. Use the nine suggested categories as a guide for overall organization.

1. Values, mission, goals
2. Education
3. Professional development
4. Professional skills
5. Professional presentations
6. Professional publications
7. Service
8. Expressions of support
9. Personal

Displaying

Finally, you must display the information you have so carefully collected, selected, and organized. Once you have all of your general information select-ed and filed by category, select one of these to begin looking at more closely for display. Neophytes often find it helpful to begin with the section on education. It is the most cut-and-dry of the sections with most of the information being official documents and certificates of achievement. It allows you to experiment with various layout methods and materials. Don't be afraid to add artifacts you previously rejected or remove something that may have seemed perfect the first time through. Use large enough print so that the viewer can get a feel for the information quickly. Remember that you do not have to have a page to display every skill and experience. Many skills, such as organizational ability, neatness, orderliness, clarity, and style, can be displayed indirectly via your overall presentation.

At this point, your portfolio should become a matter of personal style and an expression of you. Choose color schemes to carry throughout the section and when laying out your pages make them pleasing to the eye. Do items balance? Can you easily get the point of the information presented? Because you may be changing items over time, be sure to use design elements and themes that can be easily reproduced. One particularly elegant portfolio used plain vellum paper but the author included something gold on each page; a sticker, a stripe, a flower. The accents were small, but striking.

Throughout the development process and again when you are finished, it is advisable to ask several people with varying backgrounds to review and critique your work. Remember, only have those that you trust view your work, especially while you are refining it. When you feel that it is finished to your satisfaction, do a small pilot showing to test its accuracy and effectiveness in portraying you and your abilities. You may wish to use the peer evaluation tools found in Section 3 to obtain feedback.

Personal Application Guide

Organizing Your Portfolio

1. Place a check in the box next to each section title you are planning on including in your portfolio. Use the blank lines to include any of your own section titles, if needed.

2. Below each section, start brainstorming about what you might want to include in each. Place parentheses around those activities that you have not yet completed but plan on accomplishing before completing your portfolio.

❑ Values, mission, goals

❑ Education

❑ Professional development

❑ Professional skills

❑ Professional presentations

❑ Professional publications

❑ Community and professional service

❑ Expressions of support

❑ Personal

❑ _____

❑ _____

Personal Application Guide

Organizing Your Portfolio: Sample Response

✓ Values, mission, goals
- Personal mission statement
- Professional mission statement

- List of important goals accomplished and future goals
-

✓ Education
- Diploma, pictures of graduation
- Transcripts

- Brief descriptions of classes
-

✓ Professional development
- 2000, 2001, 2003 AOTA conferences I attended; pictures and descriptions of workshops and certificates

- List of local and state conferences I attended
- Professional memberships that I maintain

✓ Professional skills
- Assessments with which I am familiar
- Documentation examples

- Physical agent modalities training and experience
-

✓ Professional publication
- AJOT article I wrote
- Local newspaper article I wrote

- Contributed chapter to Ultrasound: Benefits & Uses
-

✓ Professional Presentations
- "PNF—The Basics," MOTA Convention 1998
- "Physical Agent Modalities Research," AOTA 2000

- "Improving Documentation Communication," 2004

✓ Community and professional service
- Wheelchair basketball tournament
- Red Cross volunteer work

- (Ramp building for needy families)
-

✓ Expressions of support
- Letter—parent of child from "play and say" group
- Letter—reference from my psychology professor

- Card—patient in rehab clinic
-

❑ Personal Information
-
-

-
-

✓ Leadership and teamwork
- President of student organization
- Treasurer of honors student organization

- Member of community outreach committee at work
-

Sample Portfolio Pages

Table of Contents

Table of Contents
Jennifer K. Sequin

I. Introduction
  • Resume
II. Education
  • Scholarships
  • Occupational Therapy Course Descriptions
  • Academic Awards
  • Transcripts
  • Diploma
  • Certification
III. Professional Development
  • Conferences Attended
IV. Professional Publications
V. Professional Presentations
VI. Professional Skills
  • Clinical Experiences
  • Occupational Therapy Externship
  • Class Projects
  • List of Assessments Administered
  • Clientele Information
VII. Service
  • Professional
  • Community
VIII. Expressions of Support

A table of contents helps show organization in your portfolio. It also acts as a good point of reference for anyone looking through your portfolio so that they can easily maneuver through the pages.

The table of contents tends to be the most simplistic. You can be as creative as you want to be: add colors, pictures, different font styles, etc. Just be sure that it is clear, concise, and easy to view.

Table of Contents

Mission Statement

Academics

Professional Development

Professional Presentations & Publications

Research

Professional Skills

Clinical Experience

Leadership & Teamwork

Community Service

Letters of Support

Sample Portfolio Pages

Section Cover Pages

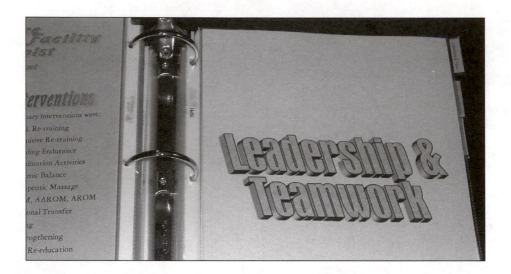

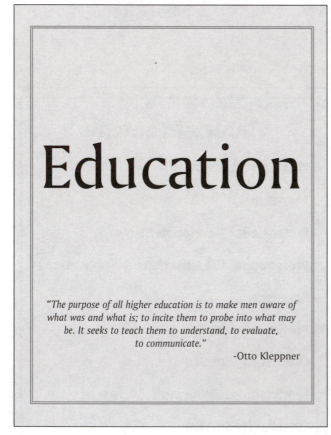

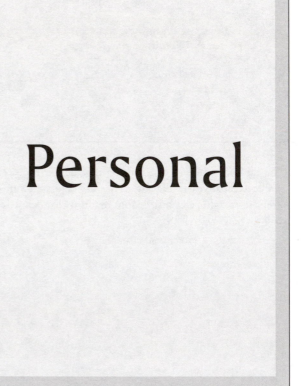

At the beginning of each section, you should have a cover page to introduce the material to follow. Remember, each page should be a reflection of you and your style.

Sample Portfolio Page

One-Page Layout

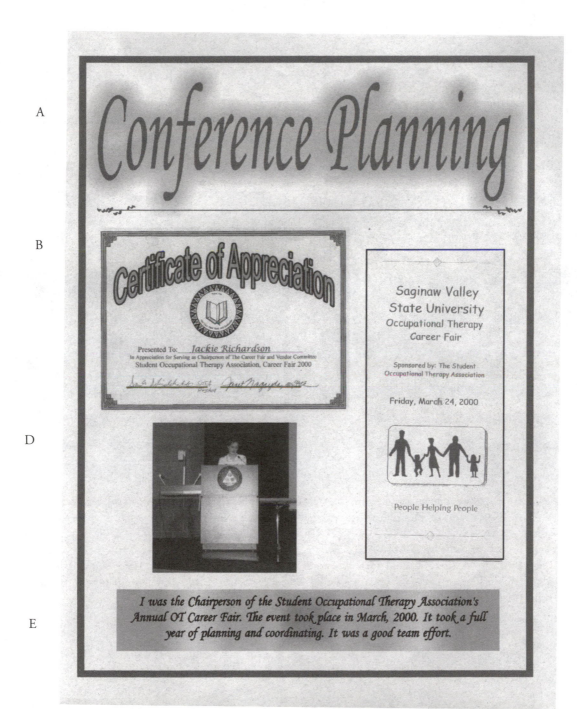

A. A concise, easy to read title is key. B. A certificate is a nice visual to demonstrate a skill or experience. C. A scanned image of a brochure adds important information in an interesting way. D. Remember, a picture says a thousand words. This photo allows people to visualize you in action. E. A shaded text box draws the eye to a brief description of the skills being demonstrated by the photos.

Sample Portfolio Pages

Two-Page Layout

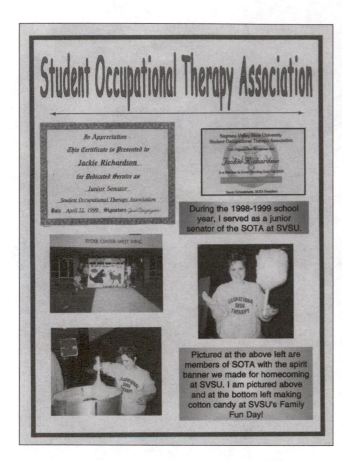

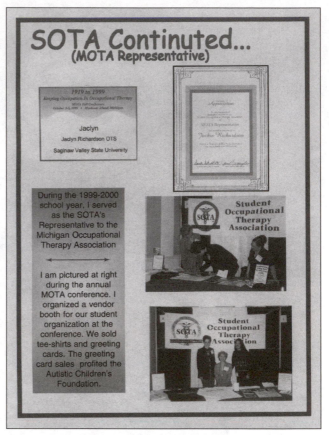

This topic requires two pages to adequately demonstrate the experiences and skills acquired when Jackie was in leadership positions with SOTA. While there are a lot of artifacts and descriptions on these pages, notice that they are not cluttered or "busy." Each artifact was chosen to draw in and show the reader a part of Jackie. For example, a copy of her SOTA membership card and a scanned image of her MOTA badge give a certain level of credibility and validity to her accomplishments. The pictures of her with cotton candy show that she is upbeat and has fun when she works. She is showing leadership and responsibility in the pictures of her going over paperwork at the vendor booth. These visuals are designed to spark interest and discussion when viewing the portfolio. Indirectly, the design of the pages display that she is organized, neat, and detail oriented.

Sample Portfolio Pages

List Format

Often, a list format is very useful and effective. There are a variety of areas that may lend themselves to lists and various ways to add some visual flair.

Academic Papers & Presentations

Papers

Case Study - CVA
Case Study - Developmental Delay
Case Study - Epicondylitis
Case Study - Profound Mental Retardation
Facet Syndrome
Shoulder Subluxation

Presentations

Cross-Training: Is There an OT in Your Future?
Degenerative Disc Disease
Developmental Dyspraxia
Rehab Centre: An In Depth Look at the Management Process
The Shoulder: Problems and Treatments

Brief descriptions give the reader a deeper understanding of the courses that you have completed better than if you simply listed the course names.

Occupational Therapy Course Descriptions (cont.)

Miscellaneous

- **OT 200 - Orientation to Occupational Therapy**
An introduction to occupational therapy practice, the history of the profession, current professional roles, issues and trends, the referral process, treatment sequence, ethics, liability, standards of practice. Emphasis on interviewing skills and therapeutic relationships. Clinical experience will be scheduled to offer observations and development of therapeutic skills.

- **OT 302 - Foundations in Occupational Therapy**
Integrates the concept of occupational performance with the influence of cultural and environmental demands. Includes learning theories, developmental transitions, supervision theories, performance evaluation and behavioral objectives. Emphasis on multicultural and societal factors influencing delivery of occupational therapy in rural areas and their influence on clinical reasoning. Students must successfully complete an eight (8) hour Level I fieldwork experience arranged by the instructor.

- **OT 308 - Therapeutic Use of Activities**
The role of activity to influence change in human performance, task analysis, use of activities as treatment modalities, analysis of specific activities for practical application. Emphasis on the balance of work, play, and self-maintenance necessary for wellness across the lifespan.

- **OT 330 - Professional Reasoning and Communications**
An introduction to documentation of occupational therapy services including effective oral, written, and nonverbal communication to facilitate accountability and service provision with patients and their families, occupational therapy personnel, other health care providers and the public. Also includes initial exposure to clinical documentation of testing methods for assessment and evaluation including the selection, administration, and interpretation of representative standardized and nonstandardized measures.

- **OT 400 - Transitions in Occupational Therapy Practice**
Frames of reference, models and theories used to integrate the practice of occupational therapy are studied. Examination of selected theoretical constructs used in occupational therapy practice and delivery and the integration of occupational therapy into the health care system. National and international health care and cultural issues and trends will be addressed with specific attention to ethical decision-making.

- **OT 422 - Therapeutic Adaptations and Technology**
Analysis, design and construction of adapted equipment to facilitate daily living skills in disabled, use of adaptive and augmentative technology, computers, and environmental controls, planning to restructure the setting to assist in self-care.

- **OT 430 - Clinical Research**
An examination of methods of scientific inquiry and empirical techniques with emphasis on occupational therapy. Review of the research process, problem definition, literature review, research design and data collection, analysis and interpretation and research reporting. Research evaluation and development of research proposal.

Sample Portfolio Pages

List Format

Pediatric Assessments

☆Bayley Scales of Infant Development

☆Bruininks-Oseretsky Test of Motor Proficiency (BOT)

☆DeGangi-Berk Test of Sensory Integration

☆Infant/Toddler Symptom Checklist: A Screening Tool for Parents

☆Miller Assessment for Preschoolers (MAP)

☆Peabody Developmental Motor Scales (PDMS)

☆Pediatric Evaluation of Disability Inventory (PEDI)

☆Sensory Integration History

Adding a colorful design to your title and clip art to your page can add some style and interest to your pages, attracting reader attention.

A list can be a great way to show a synopsis of your work. Stars or other bullets can denote that examples are provided in the portfolio.

Documentation

Screenings

Driving Evaluations
Pediatric Rehabilitation
Skilled Nursing Facility

Initial Evaluations

Community Mental Health
Functional Capacity Evaluation
☆ Inpatient Rehabilitation
Pediatric Rehabilitation
☆ Skilled Nursing Facility

Daily Notes

Community Mental Health
Inpatient Rehabilitation
Outpatient Rehabilitation
☆ Pediatric Rehabilitation
Skilled Nursing Facility

☆ Denotes example provided

Sample Portfolio Pages

List Format

Michigan Occupational Therapy Association (MOTA) 2000

I attended the following institutes:

* **You ARE What You Document**

   This one-day institute identified why it is important to document, discussed the function and form of effective documentation for reimbursement and taught clinicians how to document thoroughly, yet efficiently.

* **Promoting Practice and the Profession: Integrating the Guide to Occupational Therapy Practice**

   This institute discussed how to use the new Guide to Occupational Therapy as a tool to evaluate, describe, and transition practice to better meet the needs of clients in the current and future health care environments. It also described how the Guide can assist OT's with justifying and promoting their services to administrators, payers, other health care practitioners, and clients.

I attended the following workshops:

* Being an Occupational F.A.N.A.T.I.C.
   * Forecaster-Advocator-Negotiator-Adventurer-Teacher-Influencer-Collaborator
* Basic Marketing for Occupational Therapy
* MOTA Business Meeting
* Portfolios! Showcase all the Skills and Abilities of Occupational Therapy
* A Dozen Do's and Don't for Motivating Patients
* Collaboration Model of Occupational Therapy and Optometry in Vision Rehabilitation of Adults and Children
* Treating Perceptual Dysfunction
* Creating your Own Job - A Recipe Martha Stewart Doesn't Have!

When attending larger conferences, you are given the opportunity to attend a wide variety of institutes, workshops, and seminars. On this page, the institutes have a very brief summary to detail what was learned, but the shorter sessions have only the titles listed.

Sample Portfolio Pages

Table of Contents

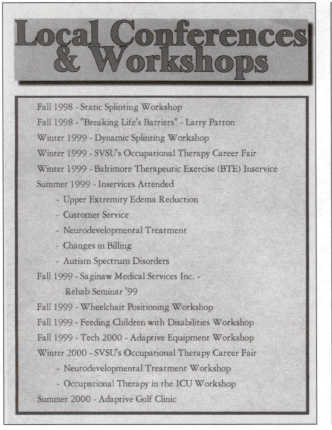

Local Conferences & Workshops

Fall 1998 - Static Splinting Workshop
Fall 1998 - "Breaking Life's Barriers" - Larry Patton
Winter 1999 - Dynamic Splinting Workshop
Winter 1999 - SVSU's Occupational Therapy Career Fair
Winter 1999 - Baltimore Therapeutic Exercise (BTE) Inservice
Summer 1999 - Inservices Attended
   - Upper Extremity Edema Reduction
   - Customer Service
   - Neurodevelopmental Treatment
   - Changes in Billing
   - Autism Spectrum Disorders
Fall 1999 - Saginaw Medical Services Inc. -
   Rehab Seminar '99
Fall 1999 - Wheelchair Positioning Workshop
Fall 1999 - Feeding Children with Disabilities Workshop
Fall 1999 - Tech 2000 - Adaptive Equipment Workshop
Winter 2000 - SVSU's Occupational Therapy Career Fair
   - Neurodevelopmental Treatment Workshop
   - Occupational Therapy in the ICU Workshop
Summer 2000 - Adaptive Golf Clinic

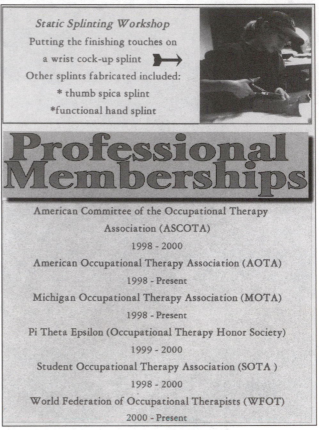

Static Splinting Workshop
Putting the finishing touches on
a wrist cock-up splint ➡
Other splints fabricated included:
* thumb spica splint
*functional hand splint

Professional Memberships

American Committee of the Occupational Therapy
Association (ASCOTA)
1998 - 2000
American Occupational Therapy Association (AOTA)
1998 - Present
Michigan Occupational Therapy Association (MOTA)
1998 - Present
Pi Theta Epsilon (Occupational Therapy Honor Society)
1999 - 2000
Student Occupational Therapy Association (SOTA)
1998 - 2000
World Federation of Occupational Therapists (WFOT)
2000 - Present

The example on the left is only a list, but you can add a picture and text box with some more details of one of the workshops from the list on the first page.

A list can have a very crisp, clean, precise feel to it. What areas in your portfolio would be expressed well with a list? How can you be creative with the lists to give them visual appeal and impact?

Sample Portfolio Pages

Tracking Sheets

Using tracking sheets in your portfolio accomplishes several goals simultaneously. First, it helps you focus on an area that you may need to improve upon, gain more experience in, or simply have an interest in. Second, it demonstrates to the viewer that you plan to continue improving in that area. Third, it gives you an easy way to track your accomplishments and education for your own records to include in your portfolio at a later time and/or to demonstrate continued competence for recertification purposes.

CONTINUING EDUCATION TRACKER

Date	Name & Location	Inservice	Workshop	Clinic	Continuing Education Credits
4-18-01	AOTA Conference: Grants: Helping OT meet the Challenge of Change		Institute		6 Contact Hours .6 CEU
4-22-01	AOTA Conference: Linking Healthy People 2010 to Diverse Populations in OT		Short Course		1.5 hours
4-22-01	AOTA Conference: Writing for AJOT: A Session with the editor		Short Course		1.5 hours

Sample Portfolio Pages

Folders

You will want to keep examples of many items easily accessible in your portfolio so that people will be able to take a closer look. This is important because having a list of skills is not the same as showing someone a tangible example of your skills. There are many ways to accomplish this. The pictures below show three ways: A) plain colored plastic folders; B) colored plastic folders with an explanation or label; or C) a simple clear sleeve protector.

A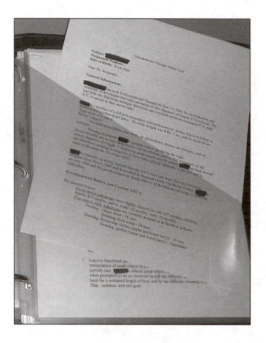

B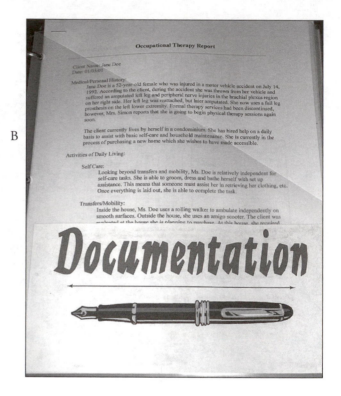

C

Sample Portfolio Pages

Folders

These are some more areas that could warrant using folders to hold examples.

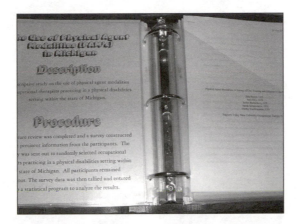

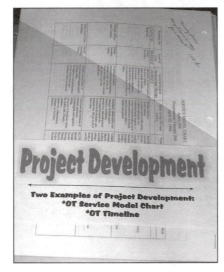

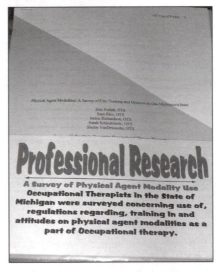

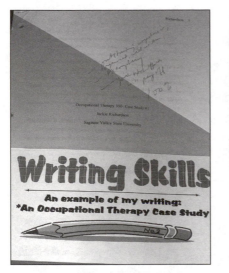

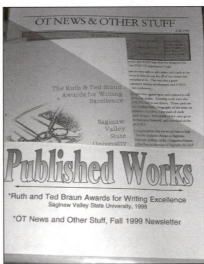

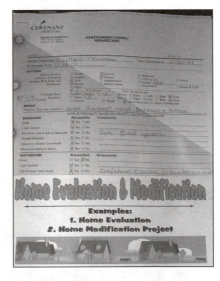

Begin Creating

Planning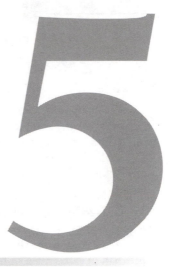

PORTFOLIO SECTIONS

The categories you select to include in your portfolio will evolve into a very personal view of your skills and experiences. It is recommended that the beginner, whether you are a student or advanced practitioner, begin with the same basic nine category headings:

1. Values, mission, and goals
2. Education
3. Professional development
4. Professional skills
5. Professional presentations
6. Professional publications
7. Service
8. Expressions of support
9. Personal

Over time, it may become appropriate to add or delete sections as your professional direction and personal interests shift. You may well need to add extra portfolio sections as you acquire specialized or nontraditional skills that may not be appropriately categorized into any of these basic sections. For example, research, leadership and management, and program development activities will all necessitate special sections. While these may seem to be more in alignment with advanced practice, practitioners at all practice levels may be involved to some degree. Students gain significant leadership and management experience through involvement in student government and other campus activities. The entry-level practitioner will look at his or her new position to see how they can make it their own. These program sections are not specific to any level of profession. When you review them, think carefully about how your own experiences may fit.

The section headings are listed in the order recommended for the portfolio content to best facilitate an understanding of your skills, experiences, and personality. You may find it helpful in the development process, however, to complete each section in the order that is easiest for you. Sections such as education and expressions of support, for example, are very different from one another and allow you to experiment with different presentation styles. This practice will be helpful to have before you tackle the more involved or less concrete sections such as the values, mission, and goals section and professional skills section. However you decide to tackle the project, remember that it can always be changed as you become more familiar with the process.

The following personal application guides are designed to help you:

* Begin to visualize your portfolio
* Determine your compelling reason to complete your portfolio
* Reflect on your strengths, skills, and areas for improvement
* Create your own definition of what being professional means
* Consider your areas of experience both in and outside of occupational therapy and how these experiences demonstrate various skills that you possess
* Think about how to demonstrate these skills in your portfolio

Personal Application Guide

Portfolio Planning

A professional portfolio can be a powerful tool for an occupational therapist. There are many different reasons to create a professional portfolio. Before you begin, think about how you are going to use your portfolio, what will need to be in it, and what steps it will take to complete it. Keep in mind that this vision for your portfolio may change along the way; this is a warm-up exercise designed to help you track your ideas.

❑ VISION: Why are you creating a professional portfolio? What are your intentions for the portfolio? What will your portfolio say about you? Identify your specific objective for the portfolio (getting a job, setting professional goals and tracking progress, tracking continuing competence, using it as a reflective process to determine current strengths and areas for improvement, showcasing your private practice or community project, recertification, etc.). You may have more than one objective, so list all that apply.

How will your portfolio support or promote the field of occupational therapy? How will it answer the question, "What is occupational therapy?"

How will your professional goals be demonstrated? How will you make them easy to identify in your portfolio?

Personal Application Guide

Portfolio Planning

❑ PHYSICAL VISION: What will your portfolio look like? What media will you use?

How your portfolio looks and presents itself says a lot about you. Some qualities do not need direct attention, but are made obvious through indirect means. Examples include neatness, organization, writing skills, and diversity. List three qualities your portfolio will indirectly say about you.

Who is your audience?

What should your audience know about you? What are your skills? Get a timer and set it for one minute. One minute is all you have to write down a list of your interpersonal skills. When the time expires, stop. Set the timer again for one minute and do the same for clinical skills and good work habits.

Interpersonal Skills	Clinical Skills	Good Work Habits

Personal Application Guide

Portfolio Planning

❏ PRACTICAL USE: Imagine taking your portfolio to a job interview and showing the finished product to the potential employer.

Name three interpersonal skills this person may look for:
    1.
    2.
    3.

> ➤ How will each be demonstrated in your portfolio?
>   1.
>   2.
>   3.

Name three clinical skills this person may look for:
    1.
    2.
    3.

> ➤ How will each be demonstrated in your portfolio?
>   1.
>   2.
>   3.

Name three good work habits this person may look for:
    1.
    2.
    3.

> ➤ How will each be demonstrated in your portfolio?
>   1.
>   2.
>   3.

❏ PLAN: Make a list of activities that you will need to do in order to complete your portfolio (no order is necessary).

Personal Application Guide
A Professional Inventory

This worksheet is designed to help you think about what being a professional means to you. It is aimed at guiding your professional development by helping you see what areas of occupational therapy excite, motivate, and drive you. It will also help you identify areas in which you need more experience.

What Makes a Person a Professional?

➤ Make a list of five professionals you find admirable. These need not be OTs, health care professionals, or even someone that you know well. For each person listed, name two things you admire about him or her.

Person	Admirable Traits
1.	
2.	
3.	
4.	
5.	

➤ Go back through the list of admirable traits you listed above and circle three or more things that you have in common with these professionals.

➤ List the traits you circled and for each trait identify a way you could display or demonstrate this attribute in your portfolio. What could you collect?

a. Admirable Trait: _____
   I could demonstrate this by _____

b. Admirable Trait: _____
   I could demonstrate this by _____

c. Admirable Trait: _____
   I could demonstrate this by _____

d. Admirable Trait: _____
   I could demonstrate this by _____

e. Admirable Trait: _____
   I could demonstrate this by _____

Personal Application Guide

A Professional Inventory

➤ Often a quality professional is one who demonstrates exceptionality and excellence. The field of occupational therapy is no exclusion to this rule. In the following space, list three to five occupational therapists and identify how each person demonstrates excellence.

1. Occupational Therapist: _____
    This person demonstrates excellence by _____
    _____

2. Occupational Therapist: _____
    This person demonstrates excellence by _____
    _____

3. Occupational Therapist: _____
    This person demonstrates excellence by _____
    _____

4. Occupational Therapist: _____
    This person demonstrates excellence by _____
    _____

5. Occupational Therapist: _____
    This person demonstrates excellence by _____
    _____

Personal Excellence

Now it is time to begin thinking about your own exceptional talents and areas of excellence. If you are a student or a beginning therapist, you may have limited direct occupational therapy experience. At this point, it becomes important to think about how you have demonstrated excellence in other areas of your life and how that can be carried into the field of occupational therapy.

➤ Identify and describe a time that you took a risk.

➤ Identify a time that you showed persistence.

➤ Name two things that your friends, family, or coworkers can count on you to be or do. How could this example be demonstrated in your portfolio? Are there pictures you could use? Are there quotes or letters of appreciation you could include?

Personal Application Guide

A Professional Inventory

➤ Another way to identify exceptional talents is by thinking about compliments people have given you. On the lines below, identify five compliments you have received.

1. _____
2. _____
3. _____
4. _____
5. _____

➤ Reflect on a time when someone asked for your help. Were you able to provide assistance? How did that person thank you, what did he or she say?

➤ List at least five exceptional talents that you possess.

Work Experience

In the space provided, make a list of the jobs and internships you have had in the last 10 years, including professional and preprofessional employment. Use another sheet of paper if necessary. For each item on your list, identify three ways in which it helped prepare you for a career in the field of occupational therapy.

Job Title	How it prepared me for occupational therapy

Personal Application Guide

A Professional Inventory

Leisure Interests

In the following space, identify your leisure interests and activities. For each item listed, document two ways this interest has prepared you for a career as an occupational therapist or has enhanced your abilities as a professional.

Interest/activity	How it prepared me for an occupational therapy career

Community Service

How, where, when, and why do you volunteer? Make a list of the service and/or volunteer activities in which you have been involved. Use additional paper if necessary.

1. _____
2. _____
3. _____
4. _____
5. _____
6. _____
7. _____
8. _____
9. _____
10. _____
11. _____
12. _____

How could you display these activities in your portfolio? What artifacts could you collect? What else could you be doing?

Personal Application Guide

A Professional Inventory

Where else could you volunteer? Think of three service projects you would like to become a part of and set a deadline for making sure you do it.

Project: _____

Deadline: _____

_____

Project: _____

Deadline: _____

_____

Project: _____

Deadline: _____

Use the following as a guide to collection of artifacts and information for your portfolio:

With whom have you worked?

What have you done?

When did you become an occupational therapy practitioner and how have you used that time?

Where have you worked, both in terms of geography and setting?

Why do you make the choices you make? (What are your professional reasoning skills and values systems?)

How did you organize your time and manage all that was required of you? How did you relate on a personal level with clients, family, coworkers, and others? Did clients feel safe with you and always feel that you were working in their best interest?

Overcoming Procrastination 6

One of the biggest hurdles in creating a portfolio is procrastination. Many people procrastinate because they feel as if they lack the time necessary to get ahead on projects. The best way to overcome this is to develop a timeline that helps you break down the process into manageable tasks with a deadline for each task. You can use a calendar, a planner, or a chart. The following personal application guide is one option to help you plan and track your progress.

Personal Application Guide

Procrastination Preventer

Week One

Goal:

Materials/support that I need to accomplish goal:

Specific tasks to be completed: Estimated time required for each task:

Schedule your time to complete each task:

Sun	Mon	Tue	Wed	Thurs	Fri	Sat

Personal Application Guide

Procrastination Preventer

Week Two

Goal:

Materials/support that I need to accomplish goal:

Specific tasks to be completed: Estimated time required for each task:

Schedule your time to complete each task:

Sun	Mon	Tue	Wed	Thurs	Fri	Sat

Personal Application Guide

Procrastination Preventer

Week Three

Goal:

Materials/support that I need to accomplish goal:

Specific tasks to be completed: Estimated time required for each task:

Schedule your time to complete each task:

Sun	Mon	Tue	Wed	Thurs	Fri	Sat

Personal Application Guide

Procrastination Preventer

Week Four

Goal:

Materials/support that I need to accomplish goal:

Specific tasks to be completed: Estimated time required for each task:

Schedule your time to complete each task:

Sun	Mon	Tue	Wed	Thurs	Fri	Sat

Personal Application Guide

Procrastination Preventer

Week Five

Goal:

Materials/support that I need to accomplish goal:

Specific tasks to be completed: Estimated time required for each task:

Schedule your time to complete each task:

Sun	Mon	Tue	Wed	Thurs	Fri	Sat

Personal Application Guide

Procrastination Preventer

Week Six

Goal:

Materials/support that I need to accomplish goal:

Specific tasks to be completed: Estimated time required for each task:

Schedule your time to complete each task:

Sun	Mon	Tue	Wed	Thurs	Fri	Sat

Personal Application Guide

Procrastination Preventer

Week Seven

Goal:

Materials/support that I need to accomplish goal:

Specific tasks to be completed: Estimated time required for each task:

Schedule your time to complete each task:

Sun	Mon	Tue	Wed	Thurs	Fri	Sat

Personal Application Guide

Procrastination Preventer

Week Eight

Goal:

Materials/support that I need to accomplish goal:

Specific tasks to be completed: Estimated time required for each task:

Schedule your time to complete each task:

Sun	Mon	Tue	Wed	Thurs	Fri	Sat

Personal Application Guide

Procrastination Preventer

Week Nine

Goal:

Materials/support that I need to accomplish goal:

Specific tasks to be completed: Estimated time required for each task:

Schedule your time to complete each task:

Sun	Mon	Tue	Wed	Thurs	Fri	Sat

Personal Application Guide

Procrastination Preventer

Week Ten

Goal:

Materials/support that I need to accomplish goal:

Specific tasks to be completed: Estimated time required for each task:

Schedule your time to complete each task:

Sun	Mon	Tue	Wed	Thurs	Fri	Sat

Personal Application Guide

Procrastination Preventer

Week Eleven

Goal:

Materials/support that I need to accomplish goal:

Specific tasks to be completed: Estimated time required for each task:

Schedule your time to complete each task:

Sun	Mon	Tue	Wed	Thurs	Fri	Sat

Personal Application Guide

Procrastination Preventer

Week Twelve

Goal:

Materials/support that I need to accomplish goal:

Specific tasks to be completed: Estimated time required for each task:

Schedule your time to complete each task:

Sun	Mon	Tue	Wed	Thurs	Fri	Sat

Section by Section

This section is designed to walk you through each section of your portfolio (what goes in each section, what skills you possess to put in each section, and samples of how to lay it all out). The format is as follows:

❋ Case study: The beginning of each section will introduce you to a different case study. Each case is fiction unless stated otherwise, so any resemblance to you or anyone that you know is purely coincidental and perhaps a little spooky. The case study will be used throughout its chapter in the completed personal application guides to demonstrate how occupational therapy practitioners at all levels of experience and in a variety of settings could use the portfolio process.

❋ Information on each specific section of the portfolio

❋ Personal application guides

❋ Collecting, selecting, organizing, and displaying chart

❋ Selecting guide

❋ Self assessment

❋ Peer assessment

❋ Sample pages

Values, Missions, and Goals

7

Case Study

Name: Doug

Age: 50

Current occupation/setting: Occupational therapy—professor at an accredited occupational therapy program

Level of experience: Experienced

Goal for portfolio: Promotion to director of occupational therapy program

This section provides the opportunity to clarify, illuminate, and state your personal and professional values, mission, and goals and reflect on your own personal belief system. What do you believe personally and professionally about the human condition, rights, and responsibilities? What is important for your audience to know about you as it relates to the purpose of your portfolio? Occupational therapy, as a profession, provides you with a place to start. Values of the profession have been articulated, which we may use to guide interactions and service provision.

CORE VALUES AND ATTITUDES

❋ Altruism: The unselfish concern for the welfare of others. This is demonstrated through commitment, caring, dedication, responsiveness, and understanding.

❋ Dignity: Emphasizes the importance of valuing the inherent worth and uniqueness of each person. This is enacted through empathy and respect for self and others.

❋ Equality: Requires that all individuals be perceived as having the same fundamental human rights and opportunities. This is demonstrated by an attitude of fairness and impartiality.

❋ Freedom: Allows individuals to exercise choice and to demonstrate independence, initiative, and self-direction.

❋ Justice: Places value on upholding moral and legal principles of fairness, equity, truthfulness, and objectivity.

❋ Truth: Requires that we be faithful to the facts and reality. You are to be accountable, honest, forthright, accurate, and authentic in attitudes and actions.

❋ Prudence: The ability to govern and discipline oneself through the use of reason. This requires judiciousness, discretion, vigilance, moderation, care, and circumspection in the management of one's affairs, the temperament of extremes, making judgments, and responding on the basis of intelligent reflection and rational thought (Kanny, 1993).

You will also want to consider intrinsic characteristics related to ethical behavior and personal honesty and integrity. *The Occupational Therapy Code of Ethics* (AOTA, 1988) provides six principles that the occupational therapy practitioner may use to guide decision making.

CODE OF ETHICS

* Beneficence: Occupational therapy personnel shall demonstrate a concern for the well being of the recipients of their services.

* Autonomy, privacy, confidentiality: Occupational therapy personnel shall respect the rights of the recipients of their services.

* Duties: Occupational therapy personnel shall achieve and continually maintain high standards of competence.

* Justice: Occupational therapy personnel shall comply with laws and Association policies guiding the profession of occupational therapy.

* Veracity: Occupational therapy personnel shall provide accurate information about occupational therapy services.

* Fidelity: Occupational therapy personnel shall treat colleagues and other professionals with fairness, discretion, and integrity.

How are all of these exemplified in your personal life and your practice? Use these to guide development of your own statement of beliefs.

MISSION STATEMENT

A mission statement, in the language of business, is an organization's basic purpose and scope of operations (Bateman & Snell, 2004). What do you want to accomplish for your clients and yourself within the context of your career? What do you need to do to meet your mission? You may think in terms of your overall view of occupational therapy or within the smallest context of practitioner/client interaction. If you find it difficult to come up with the right words to convey your thoughts, you may find it helpful to read the words of others. Review the history of occu-

Collecting, Selecting, Organizing, and Displaying

Collecting
* Review business mission statements
* Read inspirational poetry
* List things and ideas important to you
* Review occupational therapy values
* Look for quotable quotes

Selecting
* Items that reflect your beliefs
* Statements consistent with your world view
* Write your own statement of beliefs
* List your personal and professional goals

Organizing
* Be succinct

Displaying
* Display for visual impact

pational therapy and contributions of our founders. Eleanor Clarke Slagle, Charles Dutton, Susan Tracy, and others all articulated a view of occupational therapy that still echoes today (Punwar, 1994). Adolf Meyer (1992) published: "The only way to attain balance… is actual doing, actual practice, a program of wholesome living as the basis of wholesome feeling and thinking and fancy and interests." With this statement as the core of your mission, your career will reflect a commitment to occupation-based practice.

The goals portion of this section encourages you to think about where you want your career to lead you. What do you hope to accomplish? Are you looking at developing your career path in a particular direction? What are you going to do to facilitate your journey? This section will need to be developed very carefully, especially as it is reflected in a pitch book version. Your general, overall plan may not be evident in your portfolio or pitch book. You may reserve its contents for your file cabinet and only reveal those portions that are reflective of the current purpose of the portfolio and pitch book. If you are going to interview in a school setting, you may only wish to include goals related to personal and career development pertinent to that context.

Personal Application Guide

Core Values and Code of Ethics

Value	What level of importance do you place on each? Score each one from 1 to 5 (1 = not important, 5 = extremely important).	How do you rate each? Rate yourself on a scale from 1 to 5 (1 = I do not demonstrate this value, 3 = I demonstrate this value 50% of the time, 5 = I consistently demonstrate this value and make a conscious effort to improve).	Where do you want to be in the future? Use a scale from 1 to 5 (1 = I do not want to demonstrate this value, 3 = I want to demonstrate this value 50% of the time, 5 = I want to consistently demonstrate this value).
Altruism			
Dignity			
Equality			
Freedom			
Justice			
Truth			
Prudence			
Beneficence			
Autonomy			
Privacy/ confidentiality			
Duties/gain and maintain competence			
Veracity			
Fidelity			

Personal Application Guide

Personal and Professional Values

List your personal and professional values.	Score each on a scale 1 to 5 (1 = not important to me, 3 = somewhat important, 5 = very important to me).	Score each on a scale 1 to 5 (1 = not important to potential audience, 3 = somewhat important, 5 = very important to potential audience).

Finally, what are your beliefs regarding your responsibilities as a professional and employee; work skills you possess such as timeliness, neatness, organization, leadership, and teamwork; and your professional responsibilities for continuing education and lifelong learning? These should be reflective of your values with your mission and goals demonstrating a commitment to continued growth.

You may begin to list these factors in the personal application guide above, which is provided for this purpose. When you have completed your list, score each item according to its level of importance to you and its value to the expected audience. This will help you further define your choices. When this activity is completed, you will need to select a means of expressing your selected themes. A variety of literary forms are available to you, including a narrative statement, a poem, or a list of beliefs and goals. You may choose to do something visual to express yourself, such as a collage or drawing. It is also acceptable to research what others have had to say. You may find that the perfect expression already exists. With a reference to credit the author or craftsman, this may be the most satisfactory option for the beginner. The means you decide to use will be a further expression of you.

Selecting Guide

Values

In the circles, write down each achievement, skill, and/or characteristic that you want showcased in your portfolio. Next to the circles, write which artifacts you will use to demonstrate the achievement. You may not have an artifact for each achievement, so you may choose to use a list or brief description instead.

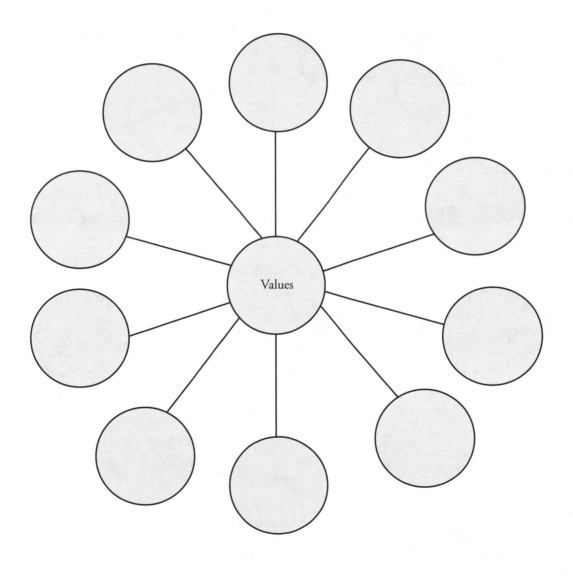

Selecting Guide

Values: Sample Response

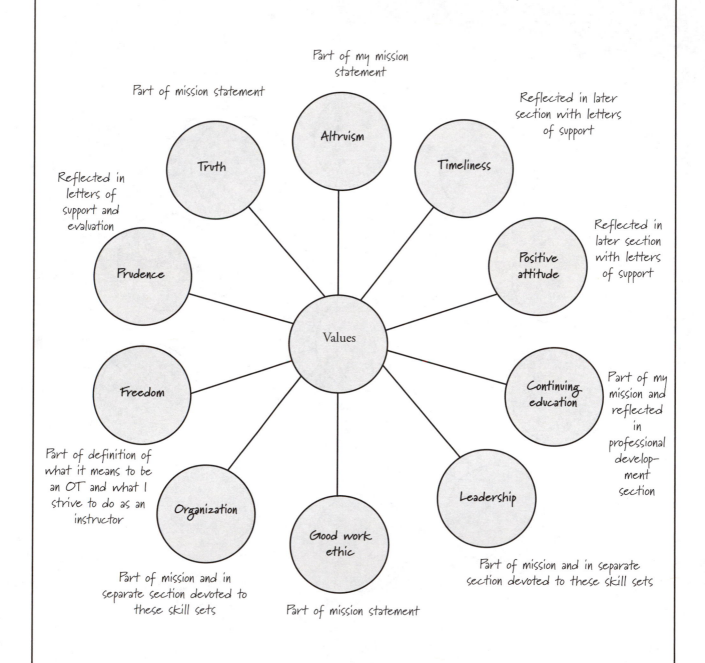

Part of my mission statement

Part of mission statement

Reflected in later section with letters of support

Altruism

Truth

Timeliness

Reflected in letters of support and evaluation

Prudence

Positive attitude

Reflected in later section with letters of support

Values

Freedom

Continuing education

Part of my mission and reflected in professional development section

Part of definition of what it means to be an OT and what I strive to do as an instructor

Organization

Good work ethic

Leadership

Part of mission and in separate section devoted to these skill sets

Part of mission and in separate section devoted to these skill sets

Part of mission statement

Self Assessment

Values, Missions, and Goals

Grade each of the categories below with a score between 1 and 5 (1 = poor, 3 = good, 5 = excellent). Feel free to make any comments you feel necessary.

Neatness	1 2 3 4 5	Comments:
Organization	1 2 3 4 5	Comments:
Completeness	1 2 3 4 5	Comments:
Content	1 2 3 4 5	Comments:
Relevancy	1 2 3 4 5	Comments:
Flow	1 2 3 4 5	Comments:
Consistency	1 2 3 4 5	Comments:
Visual appearance	1 2 3 4 5	Comments:
Representative of you	1 2 3 4 5	Comments:
Appropriate amount of info	1 2 3 4 5	Comments:

Peer Evaluation

Values, Missions, and Goals

After reviewing your peer's portfolio, grade each of the categories below with a score between 1 and 5 (1 = poor, 3 = good, 5 = excellent). Feel free to make any comments you feel necessary.

Neatness	1 2 3 4 5	Comments:
Organization	1 2 3 4 5	Comments:
Completeness	1 2 3 4 5	Comments:
Content	1 2 3 4 5	Comments:
Relevancy	1 2 3 4 5	Comments:
Flow	1 2 3 4 5	Comments:
Consistency	1 2 3 4 5	Comments:
Visual appearance	1 2 3 4 5	Comments:
Representative of you	1 2 3 4 5	Comments:
Appropriate amount of info	1 2 3 4 5	Comments:

Peer evaluator's name:

Date:

Sample Portfolio Page

Personal Vision:

To be a well rounded, competent
individual. Displaying continual
development, open mindedness, and
willingness to learn in all areas of
my life, including familial, spiritual
professional and academic.

"Keep your aspirations high enough to inspire you,
but low enough to encourage you."

-Author Unknown

Sample Portfolio Page

MISSION STATEMENT

My Personal Mission Statement:

-To gain as much knowledge as possible in every way possible
-To use this knowledge to help as many people as I can
-To enjoy something every day that God gives me
-To spend time with my friends and family
-To embrace change as a new possibility

My Professional Mission Statement:

-To use my skills effectively to help others
-To do my best in every situation
-To see what needs to be done and be sure that it gets done
-To go beyond role delineations if they prohibit me from helping someone
-To embrace change as a new opportunity

Sample Portfolio Page

Quotable Quotes

> The only way we fail
> is when we stop trying.

> The only limitations we have
> are the ones we place on ourselves.

> If you want to change the situation you first have to change yourself. And to change yourself effectively you first need to change your perceptions (Covey).

> For every thousand hacking at the leaves of evil, there is one striking at the root (Thoreau).

> It is the weak who are cruel. Gentleness can only be expected from the strong (Leo Roskin).

Sample Portfolio Page

As President I established goals to give me and the organization direction. The following are the nine goals that I set prior to beginning the term. All of these goals were discussed and ratified by the organization.

Goal 1 Met - Revise the Standard Operating Procedures

- The position descriptions were revised and updated to reflect the current responsibilities of each officer.

- The Standard Operating Procedures was discussed with suggestions made; the final revision was completed and ratified by the next class.

Goal 2 Met -Increase the number of students involved in SOTA

- We created committees with general members in charge.

- I announced every meeting time, posted the agendas prior to meetings and posted the minutes from each meeting.

Goal 3 Met - Increase junior and senior student interaction

- We sponsored two successful mentoring activities with a "buddy" system in place.

- We increased personal interaction through the "buddy" system and through a common resource center in which students could ask questions.

-Office positions often consisted of one junior and one senior student

A Saginaw Valley State University newspaper article featuring one of our student mentoring activities. ➡

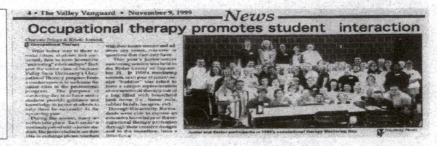

Occupational therapy promotes student interaction

Education 8

Case Study

Name: Tim

Age: 25

Current occupation/setting: OTA in an acute care setting at a local hospital

Level of experience: Entry-level

Goal for portfolio: Moving to new state and needs to find a new job

A REFLECTION

The education section of the professional portfolio is a reflection of your formal educational experience. This includes anything that supports or leads to grades and degrees. It does not include continuing education activities.

Collecting

The collection of artifacts should follow the progression of your educational history and includes any formal education and degrees you have earned, not just those in occupational therapy. These may include transcripts, scholarships, academic honors and awards, and photos of interest. It is not recommended that mention be made of your high school academics unless there is some kind of a logical trend being demonstrated and, even then, it should be very brief. Depending on your unique situation, it may also be appropriate to include extra curricular activities directly related to your educational experience, such as tutoring, international studies, and other opportunities you may have taken advantage of to operate and support your learning.

Selecting

Selecting artifacts for this section relies heavily on personal preference and situation. For example, if you are a new graduate, this may be your strongest section. Select items directly related to grades and degrees. Do not be tempted to include samples of your academic work for this section. You may, however, want to include your Level II fieldwork final evaluations in their entirety. You will also include academic and scholastic certificates and awards of achievement. The more experienced practitioner will be more concerned with selecting items to highlight their experience beyond education. This section will stand more as a summary of educational and scholastic accomplishments.

Organizing

Organization of the education section is very straightforward and concise. The most common format is to organize educational history with the most recent accomplishments first. If you attended multiple educational institutions, you will need to decide whether to keep all information for each setting together, or put information together by type (i.e., group all transcripts together, all awards together, and so on). Students and entry-level practitioners will be more likely to identify their fieldwork sites in this section, but this is not the place to discuss what happened there. Level II fieldwork final evaluations may be included here but should be placed in a pocket to keep them together. The alternate location for evaluations is in the professional skills section.

Displaying

How you choose to display these artifacts becomes a matter of personal style. Using photos of you taking part in educational activities and ceremonies personalizes the information but you will want to be careful not to interfere with the serious nature of the information. Handle important documents carefully. Don't cut up your diploma just to make it fit on a page! You may scan any of these documents and then manipulate them on the computer. The same can be done with any written artifact. If you received five certificates for being on the Dean's list, scan one of them and then write a brief list of the semesters they were awarded. This saves room and keeps the reader from looking at the same type of item over and over. If you have a multi-page document that you feel is necessary to include, place it in

Collecting, Selecting, Organizing, and Displaying

Collecting
- ✳ Transcripts
- ✳ Scholarship awards
- ✳ Academic award certificates
- ✳ Diplomas
- ✳ Photos of educational and/or extracurricular activities

Selecting
- ✳ Artifacts that represent formal educational experiences
- ✳ Items showcasing your scholastic abilities

Organizing
- ✳ According to educational history with recent first
- ✳ Use photos as long as they do not interfere with the serious nature of the information

Displaying
- ✳ Use photos as long as they do not interfere with the nature of the information

a pocket. You may also want to neatly use a highlighter to draw the reader's attention to particular information. Just make sure the display communicates the serious nature of the information.

Selecting Guide

Education

In the circles, write down each achievement, skill, and/or characteristic that you want showcased in your portfolio. Next to the circles, write which artifacts you will use to demonstrate the achievement. You may not have an artifact for each achievement, so you may choose to use a list of brief description instead.

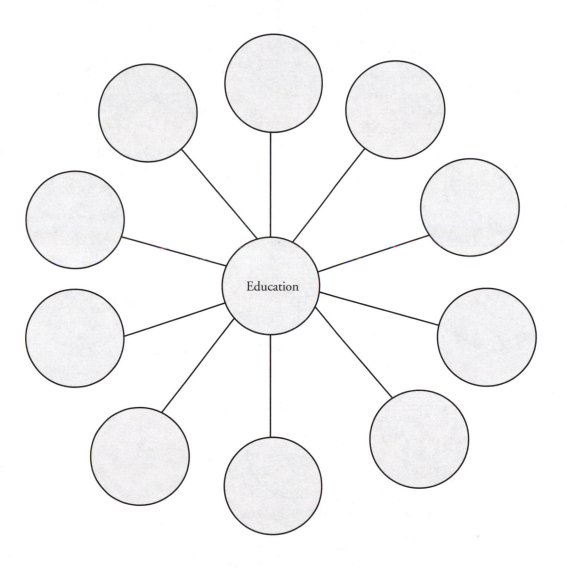

Selecting Guide

Education: Sample Response

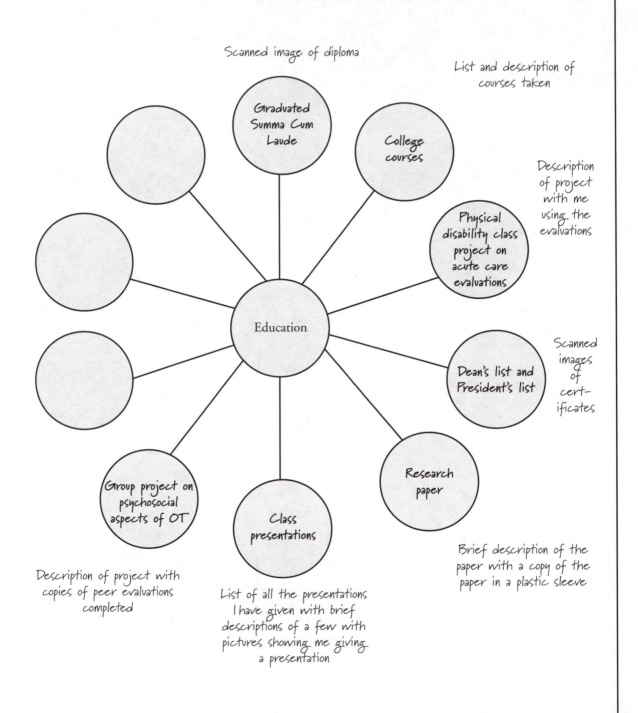

Scanned image of diploma

List and description of courses taken

Graduated Summa Cum Laude

College courses

Physical disability class project on acute care evaluations

Description of project with me using the evaluations

Education

Dean's list and President's list

Scanned images of certificates

Research paper

Group project on psychosocial aspects of OT

Class presentations

Description of project with copies of peer evaluations completed

List of all the presentations I have given with brief descriptions of a few with pictures showing me giving a presentation

Brief description of the paper with a copy of the paper in a plastic sleeve

Self Assessment

Education

Grade each of the categories below with a score between 1 and 5 (1 = poor, 3 = good, 5 = excellent). Feel free to make any comments you feel necessary.

Neatness	1 2 3 4 5	Comments:
Organization	1 2 3 4 5	Comments:
Completeness	1 2 3 4 5	Comments:
Content	1 2 3 4 5	Comments:
Relevancy	1 2 3 4 5	Comments:
Flow	1 2 3 4 5	Comments:
Consistency	1 2 3 4 5	Comments:
Visual appearance	1 2 3 4 5	Comments:
Representative of you	1 2 3 4 5	Comments:
Appropriate amount of info	1 2 3 4 5	Comments:

Peer Evaluation

Education

After reviewing your peer's portfolio, grade each of the categories below with a score between 1 and 5 (1 = poor, 3 = good, 5 = excellent). Feel free to make any comments you feel necessary.

Neatness	1 2 3 4 5	Comments:
Organization	1 2 3 4 5	Comments:
Completeness	1 2 3 4 5	Comments:
Content	1 2 3 4 5	Comments:
Relevancy	1 2 3 4 5	Comments:
Flow	1 2 3 4 5	Comments:
Consistency	1 2 3 4 5	Comments:
Visual appearance	1 2 3 4 5	Comments:
Representative of you	1 2 3 4 5	Comments:
Appropriate amount of info	1 2 3 4 5	Comments:

Peer evaluator's name:

Date:

Sample Portfolio Page

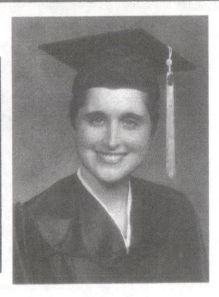

Graduated, Summa Cum Laude with a Bachelor of Science in Occupational Therapy in December 2000 from Saginaw Valley State University

Saginaw Valley State University

On recommendation of the Faculty, and by authority of the State of Michigan, the Board of Control has conferred the Degree

Bachelor of Science

summa cum laude

upon

Jaclyn M. Richardson

who has fulfilled all requirements for the Degree and is entitled to all rights and privileges pertaining thereto.

Given at University Center, Michigan, this

15th day of December, 2000

President of the University

Chairman of the Board of Control

Sample Portfolio Page

Educational History

Secondary Education

Brown City High School, Brown City, Michigan
Graduated in May, 1995

College Education

Calvin College, Grand Rapids, Michigan
Attended August 1995 to May 1997

Saginaw Valley State University
Attended August 1997 to December 2000
Graduated, December 2000
Major in Occupational Therapy
Minor in Psychology

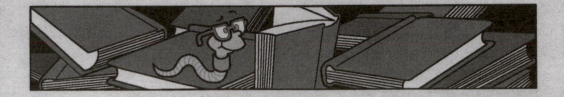

─── **Sample Portfolio Page** ───

President's List
Saginaw Valley State University

SAGINAW VALLEY STATE UNIVERSITY

This is to certify that the Registrar,
authorized by the President of the University,
has recorded the name of

Jaclyn M Hill

on the
PRESIDENT'S LIST
in recognition of the highest academic achievement
for the Fall 1997 semester.

Fall Semester, 1997

SAGINAW VALLEY STATE UNIVERSITY

This is to certify that the Registrar,
authorized by the President of the University,
has recorded the name of

Jaclyn M Hill

on the
PRESIDENT'S LIST
in recognition of the highest academic achievement
for the Winter 1998 semester.

Winter Semester, 1998

SAGINAW VALLEY STATE UNIVERSITY

This is to certify that the Registrar,
authorized by the President of the University,
has recorded the name of

Jaclyn M Richardson

on the
PRESIDENT'S LIST
in recognition of the highest academic achievement
for the Fall 1998 semester.

Fall Semester, 1998

SAGINAW VALLEY STATE UNIVERSITY

This is to certify that the Registrar,
authorized by the President of the University,
has recorded the name of

Jaclyn M Richardson

on the
PRESIDENT'S LIST
in recognition of the highest academic achievement
for the Winter 1999 semester.

Winter Semester, 1999

SAGINAW VALLEY STATE UNIVERSITY

This is to certify that the Registrar,
authorized by the President of the University,
has recorded the name of

Jaclyn M Richardson

on the
PRESIDENT'S LIST
in recognition of the highest academic achievement
for the Fall 1999 semester.

Fall Semester, 1999

SAGINAW VALLEY STATE UNIVERSITY

This is to certify that the Registrar,
authorized by the President of the University,
has recorded the name of

Jaclyn M Richardson

on the
PRESIDENT'S LIST
in recognition of the highest academic achievement
for the Winter 2000 semester.

Winter Semester, 2000

Sample Portfolio Page

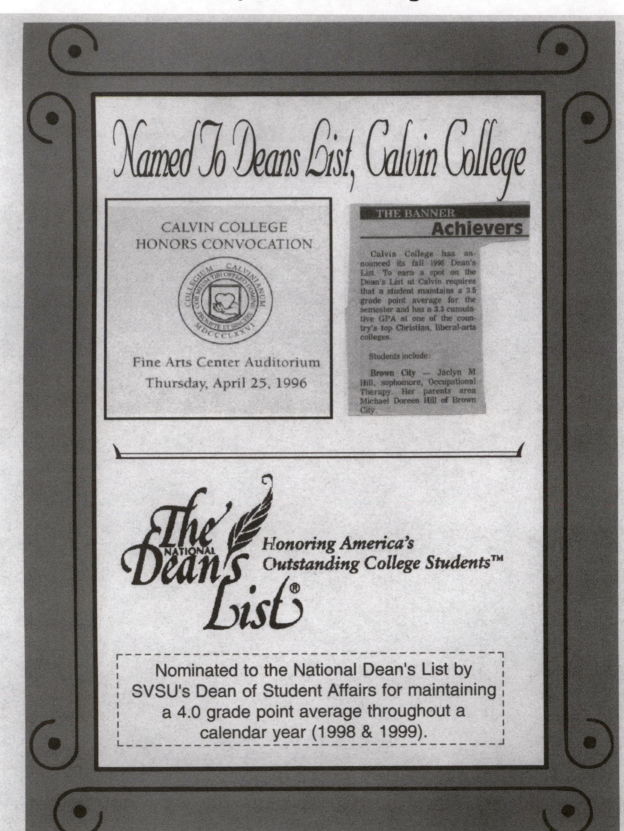

Named To Deans List, Calvin College

CALVIN COLLEGE HONORS CONVOCATION

Fine Arts Center Auditorium
Thursday, April 25, 1996

THE BANNER
Achievers

Calvin College has announced its fall 1996 Dean's List. To earn a spot on the Dean's List at Calvin requires that a student maintains a 3.5 grade point average for the semester and has a 3.3 cumulative GPA at one of the country's top Christian, liberal-arts colleges.

Students include:

Brown City — Jaclyn M Hill, sophomore, Occupational Therapy. Her parents area Michael Doreen Hill of Brown City.

The NATIONAL Dean's List®
Honoring America's Outstanding College Students™

Nominated to the National Dean's List by SVSU's Dean of Student Affairs for maintaining a 4.0 grade point average throughout a calendar year (1998 & 1999).

Sample Portfolio Page

Academic Awards

VICE PRESIDENT OF INSTRUCTION AND LEARNING SERVICES

Delta College
We Are Your Opportunity

March 8, 2000

Jennifer Kay Scoles
2918 W River Rd
Midland, MI 48642

Dear Ms. Scoles:

It is with pleasure that I notify you that your scholarly achievement, as indicated by a GPA of 3.908 for the Fall 1999 Semester, has entitled you to be placed on the Vice President's List for outstanding academic performance. Your record not only reflects very favorably on you but brings honor to Delta College in its quest for educational excellence.

I extend to you my heartiest congratulations and hope that you will continue to maintain your notable position among Delta's student body.

Sincerely,

Betty B. Jones

Betty B. Jones, Ph.D.
Vice President of Instruction and Learning Services

mra

Delta College Vice President's List
(3.7 - 3.99 grade point average for semester)
Spring 1999
Fall 1999
Winter 2000

SAGINAW VALLEY STATE UNIVERSITY

This is to certify that the Registrar,
authorized by the President of the University,
has recorded the name of

Jennifer K Scoles

on the

PRESIDENT'S LIST

in recognition of the highest academic achievement
for the Fall 2000 semester.

REGISTRAR   PRESIDENT

SVSU President's List
(4.0 grade point average for semester)
Fall 2000
Winter 2001
Spring 2001
Fall 2001
Winter 2002
Fall 2002
Winter 2003

Sample Portfolio Page

Occupational Therapy Course Descriptions

Physical Disabilities

- **OT 326 - Conditions and Approaches to Orthopedics**
  A study of the orthopedic conditions encountered by occupational therapists. Etiology, assessment, management and treatment of orthopedic conditions are studied. Clinical experience presenting functional treatment approaches to orthopedic conditions, emphasis on hand evaluation, treatment, and splinting.

- **OT 328 - Conditions and Approaches to Physical Dysfunction**
  Musculoskeletal, neurological and neuromuscular systems are studied with selected physical conditions including etiology, symptoms, and functional deficits resulting from disease or injury treated in occupational therapy practice. Emphasis on normal and abnormal function over the lifespan.

- **OT 350 - Occupational Therapy Treatment of Physical Disabilities**
  Evaluation and basic treatment for neurology, orthopedic, traumatic and degenerative conditions; current theories and concepts of occupational therapy intervention; application of occupational therapy treatment approaches to specific disabilities. Experiential learning in health care facilities will be included.

Psychosocial Dysfunction

- **OT 420 - Conditions and Approaches to Psychosocial Dysfunction**
  Review of the etiology, symptomatology and functional sequelae of major psychiatric disorders treated in occupational therapy practice. Review of psychopathology, theoretical frames of reference, evaluation, treatment and management of psychiatric and developmentally disabling conditions.

- **OT 440 - Occupational Therapy Treatment of Psychosocial Dysfunction**
  The study of principles of psychiatric occupational therapy practice in the evaluation and treatment of individuals with developmental disabilities or psychosocial dysfunction. Review of psychopathology and theoretical frames of reference in occupational therapy intervention and treatment. Experiential learning will be scheduled in occupational therapy mental health and various community treatment programs.

Pediatrics

- **OT 410 - Conditions and Approaches in Pediatric Occupational Therapy**
  Theories and principles of evaluation and therapeutic intervention for clients from birth to age 18; emphasis on growth and development, congenital and acquired conditions of childhood, educational terminology, roles and functions of the occupational therapists in educational settings are examined.

Listing and giving a brief description of your academic courses can give the audience a clearer understanding of what you learned in school.

You can organize this list in a variety of ways, as long as it makes sense to you and seems logical to others. Here are two examples. The top sample lists the courses according to the area of practice to which each pertains. The sample to the right lists each course in the order taken. Which way do you prefer? Or do you have another choice?

Summary of Educational Curriculum

Professional Occupational Therapy Coursework

OT 200   Orientation to Occupational Therapy
- An introduction to occupational therapy practice, the history of the profession, current professional roles, issues and trends, the referral process, treatment sequence, ethics, liability and standards of practice.

OT 302   Foundations in Occupational Therapy
- Integrates the concept of occupational performance with the influence of cultural and environmental demands. Includes learning theories, developmental transitions, supervision theories, performance evaluation and behavioral objectives.

OT 308   Therapeutic Use of Activities
- The role of activity to influence change in human performance: task analysis, use of activities as treatment modalities, analysis of specific activities for practical application.

OT 326   Conditions and Approaches to Orthopedics
- Etiology, assessment, management and treatment of orthopedic conditions are studied. Clinical experience presenting functional treatment approaches to orthopedic conditions, emphasis on hand evaluation, treatment and splinting.

OT 328   Conditions and Approaches to Physical Dysfunction
- Musculo-skeletal, neurological and neuro-muscular systems are studied with selected physical conditions including etiology, symptoms and functional deficits resulting from disease or injury treated in occupational therapy practice.

OT 330   Professional Reasoning & Communication
- An introduction to documentation of occupational therapy services including effective oral, written and non-verbal communication to facilitate accountability and service provision. Includes initial exposure to clinical documentation of testing methods for assessment and evaluation including the selection, administration and interpretation of representative standardized and non-standardized measures.

OT 350   Occupational Therapy Treatment of Physical Disabilities
- Evaluation and basic treatment for neurology, orthopedic, traumatic and degenerative conditions; current theories and concepts of occupational therapy intervention; application of occupational therapy treatment approaches to specific disabilities.

OT 400   Transitions in Occupational Therapy Practice
- Frames of reference, models and theories used to integrate the practice of occupational therapy are studied. Examination of selected theoretical constructs used in occupational therapy practice and delivery and the integration of occupational therapy into the health care system. National and international health care and cultural issues and trends are addressed with specific attention to ethical decision making.

Sample Portfolio Page

Class Projects

- **Adaptive Toy/Switch**

  In our Therapeutic Adaptations and Technology in OT class we each constructed a copper wafer adapter (aka a "pigtail"), permanently adapted a battery-operated toy, and fabricated an adaptive lever push switch. (The picture below taken at the Millet Learning Center, shows a young girl with cerebral palsy mixing up some chocolate milk using my adapted Easy Bake Blender and switch.)

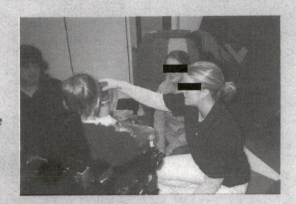

- **Disability Awareness Project**

  In our Professional Reasoning and Communication class we were each given several disabilities that we had to emulate as we shopped in Meijers. We were given a list of things to do including asking an employee for help, trying on a piece of clothing, and purchasing one small item. I emulated an *obese* individual whom had a CVA on the right side with a glenohumeral subluxation and Broca's aphasia. This assignment helped me to realize what the client is going through and what it feels like to have several disabilities.

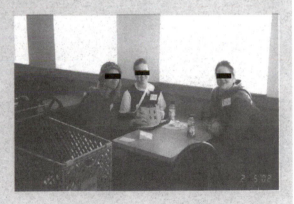

- **Community Project**

  Also in our Therapeutic Adaptations and Technology in OT class we were given the assignment of partaking in a community project of our choice. I chose to mentor a freshman student on campus who had Asperger's Syndrome. We met once a week for approximately an hour to discuss his organization, and any difficulties he was having on campus, in the classroom, or socially. At the end of one semester the student reported feeling more organized and morecomfortable with campus operations. The student also felt that he was better familiarized with all the resources SVSU's campus has to offer.

Sample Portfolio Page

Academic Papers & Presentations

Papers

Shoulder Subluxation

Facet Syndrome

Case Study- Epicondylitis

Case Study - CVA

Case Study - Developmental Delay

Case Study - Profound Mental Retardation

Papers & Presentations

Degenerative Disc Disease

Developmental Dyspraxia

Cross-Training - Is there an OT in Your Future?

The Shoulder - Problems and Treatments

RehabCentre - An Indepth Look at the

Management Process

Professional Development

9

Case Study

Name: Emily

Age: 25

Current occupation/setting: OTA in inpatient rehab center

Level of experience: Intermediate

Goal for portfolio: Wants to transition into new career at hand clinic

---

BEYOND EDUCATION

This section highlights those learning activities you have engaged in to develop your knowledge and skill base beyond the formal academic setting. This will be especially relevant for the intermediate and advanced practitioner as well as the re-entry practitioner. The entry-level practitioner may not have had sufficient time to engage in very many of these activities, but it is important that he or she shows that he or she values these experiences and plan to seek out opportunities to engage in them as they become necessary and available in the future.

Collecting

The collection of artifacts related to continuing education activities requires the development of a method to keep track of all the relevant information. You will undoubtedly bring home brochures, handouts, and notes taken from continuing education activities, as well as a certificate verifying participation. File these things together for later retrieval. It

can be developed to reflect the various requirements of applicable accrediting bodies. You will also want to discover whether your employer will require this type of information and build in the necessary charting data. It may also be helpful to consider the possibility of a specialty certification or other advanced recognition in your future. The application process for advanced recognition often considers past activities you have been engaged in and you will need to be able to lay your hands on this proof of attendance and accomplishment.

Selecting

Selecting the appropriate information for inclusion in your portfolio is fairly easy in this section. The portfolio can handle a summary of all the continuing education activities in which you engage. This may include the original charting system. You need to decide the type of impact you wish to make. Do you want to bowl them over with the extent of your activities, or do you want to zero in on a particular type of experience? How much do they need to know about the content? A list may be sufficient, but it may be more illuminating and interesting, to include the occasional brochure, outline of content, and picture.

Organizing

Organizing these disparate information types may be done in several ways. The first is to just include your charting as it develops. Some people choose a handwritten method, but is this what you want the reader to see? If may be more efficient to keep a running chart on your computer so you can download the most current version at will. It certainly will provide a better looking, more professional document. The charts may give a chronological view of your advanced learning activities or they may be organized according to subject matter. The choice will reflect your purpose.

The second organizational method is to include artifacts that highlight particularly relevant continuing education opportunities or professional development activities that will enhance your value to the reader. The important point here is to not overdo it. Don't swamp the reader in artifacts or he or she will loose the connection to the information.

Displaying

The display of information in this section needs to promote an interest in the reviewer but should not overpower the content. The reviewer should be led to the conclusion that you take the development of your professional knowledge and skills very seriously and intend to continue. Artifacts that demonstrate

your ability to apply the information learned should certainly be included. These may include sample treatment plans, pictures of you and your clients, or pictures of items such as splints that you have fabricated based on the information learned.

Collecting, Selecting, Organizing, and Displaying

Collecting
* Attendance confirmations
* Brochures
* Pictures of you at the presentation and applying the information and skills

Selecting
* Verification of attendance
* Artifacts showing your application of selected information and skills

Organizing
* Most recent continuing education activity first
* Organize according to date
* May also be divided according to content area

Displaying
* An easy to see overview of continuing education accomplishments
* Pictures to promote interest

Selecting Guide

Professional Development

In the circles, write down each achievement, skill, and/or characteristic that you want showcased in your portfolio. Next to the circles, write which artifacts you will use to demonstrate the achievement. You may not have an artifact for each achievement, so you may choose to use a list of brief description instead.

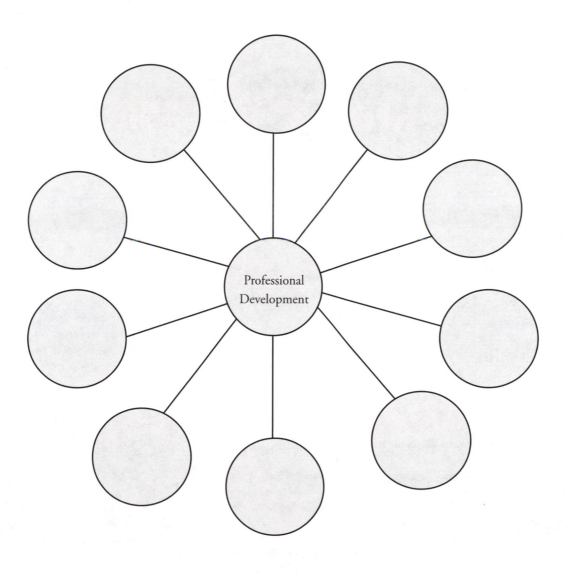

Selecting Guide

Professional Development: Sample Response

List and description of
each inservice with
tracking sheet for
future inservices

List of clients, diagnoses,
goals, and treatment plans

List of organizations and
time I have been a
member

Pictures of me
creating variety
of splints; copy
of certificate
of completion

Details of my
volunteer work
and pictures

**Inservices
attended at
work**

**Clients,
diagnoses, and
treatments**

**Professional
memberships**

**Volunteer
work at hand
clinic**

**Splinting
workshop**

Professional
Development

**Guest lecture
at local
university**

**Attended state
conference
workshop on
hand injuries**

Pictures of me
speaking/interacting
with students; brief
description of topic

**Group study on
wound care and
healing process**

**Completed self
study course on
carpal tunnel**

**Attended
AOTA's
conference**

Pictures of me
participating
with brief
description

Brief summary of how we conducted
group, goals, accomplishments, and how
it all affected me; pictures of group
interaction

Scan certificate of
completion

Complete list of events, seminars,
workshops, and poster sessions
attended; scan certificate of
completion.

Self Assessment

Professional Development

After reviewing your portfolio, grade each of the categories below with a score between 1 and 5 (1 = poor, 3 = good, 5 = excellent). Feel free to make any comments you feel necessary.

Neatness	1 2 3 4 5	Comments:
Organization	1 2 3 4 5	Comments:
Completeness	1 2 3 4 5	Comments:
Content	1 2 3 4 5	Comments:
Relevancy	1 2 3 4 5	Comments:
Flow	1 2 3 4 5	Comments:
Consistency	1 2 3 4 5	Comments:
Visual appearance	1 2 3 4 5	Comments:
Representative of you	1 2 3 4 5	Comments:
Appropriate amount of info	1 2 3 4 5	Comments:

Peer Evaluation

Professional Development

After reviewing your peer's portfolio, grade each of the categories below with a score between 1 and 5 (1 = poor, 3 = good, 5 = excellent). Feel free to make any comments you feel necessary.

Neatness	1 2 3 4 5	Comments:
Organization	1 2 3 4 5	Comments:
Completeness	1 2 3 4 5	Comments:
Content	1 2 3 4 5	Comments:
Relevancy	1 2 3 4 5	Comments:
Flow	1 2 3 4 5	Comments:
Consistency	1 2 3 4 5	Comments:
Visual appearance	1 2 3 4 5	Comments:
Representative of you	1 2 3 4 5	Comments:
Appropriate amount of info	1 2 3 4 5	Comments:

Peer evaluator's name:

Date:

Sample Portfolio Page

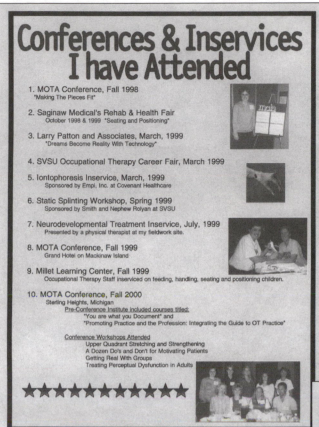

Conferences & Inservices I have Attended

1. MOTA Conference, Fall 1998
"Making The Pieces Fit"

2. Saginaw Medical's Rehab & Health Fair
October 1998 & 1999 "Seating and Positioning"

3. Larry Patton and Associates, March, 1999
"Dreams Become Reality With Technology"

4. SVSU Occupational Therapy Career Fair, March 1999

5. Iontophoresis Inservice, March, 1999
Sponsored by Empi, Inc. at Covenant Healthcare

6. Static Splinting Workshop, Spring 1999
Sponsored by Smith and Nephew Rolyan at SVSU

7. Neurodevelopmental Treatment Inservice, July, 1999
Presented by a physical therapist at my fieldwork site.

8. MOTA Conference, Fall 1999
Grand Hotel on Mackinaw Island

9. Millet Learning Center, Fall 1999
Occupational Therapy Staff inserviced on feeding, handling, seating and positioning children.

10. MOTA Conference, Fall 2000
Sterling Heights, Michigan
Pre-Conference Institute included courses titled:
"You are what you Document" and
"Promoting Practice and the Profession: Integrating the Guide to OT Practice"

Conference Workshops Attended
Upper Quadrant Stretching and Strengthening
A Dozen Do's and Don't for Motivating Patients
Getting Real With Groups
Treating Perceptual Dysfunction in Adults

★★★★★★★★★★★★★

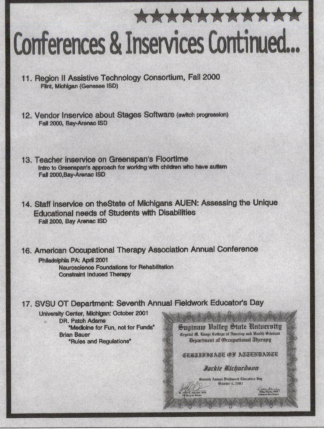

★★★★★★★★★★★★★

Conferences & Inservices Continued...

11. Region II Assistive Technology Consortium, Fall 2000
Flint, Michigan (Genesee ISD)

12. Vendor Inservice about Stages Software (switch progression)
Fall 2000, Bay-Arenac ISD

13. Teacher Inservice on Greenspan's Floortime
Intro to Greenspan's approach for working with children who have autism
Fall 2000, Bay-Arenac ISD

14. Staff inservice on the State of Michigans AUEN: Assessing the Unique Educational needs of Students with Disabilities
Fall 2000, Bay Arenac ISD

16. American Occupational Therapy Association Annual Conference
Philadelphia PA: April 2001
Neuroscience Foundations for Rehabilitation
Constraint Induced Therapy

17. SVSU OT Department: Seventh Annual Fieldwork Educator's Day
University Center, Michigan: October 2001
DR. Patch Adams
"Medicine for Fun, not for Funds"
Brian Bauer
"Rules and Regulations"

Sample Portfolio Page

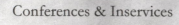

Conferences & Inservices

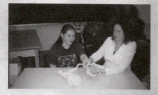

December 2000
- Splint Workshop at Saginaw Valley State University with Sammons and Preston

September 2000
- Wheelchair inservice by Saginaw Medical

October 2001
- Grants and proposals inservice

October 2001
- Wheelchair Seating and Positioning Workshop at the Millet Learning Center

---

November 2001
- Augmentative Communication and Assistive Technology Workshop at the Millet Learning Center

November 2001
- Reflexes and Reactions – Positioning and Handling Workshop at the Millet Learning Center

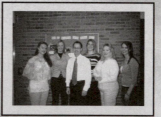

October 2001
- Patch Adams Conference at Saginaw Valley State University

November 2001
- Adaptive Seating Workshop at Saginaw Valley State University

November 2001
- Feeding Workshop at the Millet Learning Center

Sample Portfolio Page

Static Splinting Workshop

Putting the finishing touches on

a wrist cock-up splint ➤

Other splints fabricated included:

* thumb spica splint

*functional hand splint

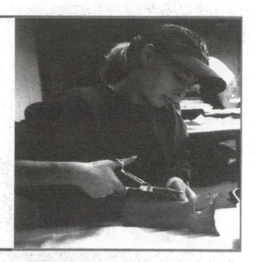

Professional Memberships

American Committee of the Occupational Therapy
Association (ASCOTA)

1998 - 2000

American Occupational Therapy Association (AOTA)

1998 - Present

Michigan Occupational Therapy Association (MOTA)

1998 - Present

Pi Theta Epsilon (Occupational Therapy Honor Society)

1999 - 2000

Student Occupational Therapy Association (SOTA)

1998 - 2000

World Federation of Occupational Therapists (WFOT)

2000 - Present

Sample Portfolio Page

Summary of Patient/Client Contacts

Staff Occupational Therapist: RehabCare at Covenant HealthCare

Ages: 16Years to 98 Years

Diagnoses: CVA, TBI, MS, Parkinson's Dementia, Vertigo Multiple Trauma Total Knee Replacement, Total Hip Replacement Shoulder Replacement, Bone Fracture, Spinal Stenosis, Deconditioning, CP, Mental Retardation with acute injury.

Level Two Fieldwork: Bay-Arenac Intermediate School District

Ages: 6 weeks to 25 years

Diagnoses: Seizure Disorder, Cerebral Palsy, Closed Head Injury, Schinzel-Gideons Syndrome, Down's Syndrome, Developmental Delay, Sensory Modulation Disorder, Visual Impairments, Learning Disability

Level Two Fieldwork and Student Extern: Gratiot Comm. Hospital

Ages: 45 Years to 78 Years

Diagnoses: CVA, Multiple Sclerosis, Traumatic Brain Injury, Crainiotomy, Parkinson's Disease, Upper and Lower Extremity Fracture, Joint Replacement, OsteoArthritis, Rheumatoid Arthritis, Diabetes, Failure to Thrive, Alzheimer's

Level One Fieldwork: Covenant Healthcare

Ages: 15 months to 74 Years

Diagnoses: Upper Extremity Fracture, Burn, Brachial Plexus Injury,   Joint Replacement, Tendon Laceration, Carpal TunnelSyndrome, DeQuarvains, Lateral Epicondylitis, Sprain, Cerebral Palsy, CVA, Craniotomy

Level One Fieldwork: Pinecrest Farms

Ages: 21 Years to 84 Years

Diagnoses: Schizophrenia, Personality Disorder, Bipolar Disorder, Depression, Anxiety Disorder, Obsessive Compulsive Disorder,   Cerebral Palsy,CVA, Closed Head Injury, Seizure Disorder

Sample Portfolio Page

Huron Memorial Hospital Outpatient Rehabilitation Level 1 Fieldwork
Jan. 1999 - April 1999

Diagnoses

→ Alzheimers
→ Below the Knee Amputation
→ CVA- Left, Right, Bilateral
→ Diabetes
→ Dementia
→ Epicondylitis
→ Rheumatoid Arthritis
→ Fractures - (simple and comminuted) radius, phalanx, hip
→ Frostbite
→ Generalized Weakness
→ Hand Injuries
  → DIP Amputation
  → Torn Cartilage
  → Volar Plate Strain
  → Finger Reattachment
  → Crush Injury
→ Hip Replacement
→ Lumbar Laminectomy
→ Post Polio Syndrome
→ Reflex Sympathetic Disorder (RSD)

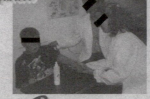

Patients

The patients ranged in age from 18 months to 100 years. The majority of the patients were adults with work or accident related injuries and older adults who suffered from CVA's.

Interventions

The most frequently used interventions:

Modalities - whirlpool, ultrasound, hot pack, iontophoresis, paraffin, NMES, static and dynamic splinting.

Therapeutic activities and exercise, therapeutic massage, AROM, AAROM, PROM and desensitization.

Personal Independence Center Community Mental Health Level 1 Fieldwork
Jan. 2000 - Apr. 2000

Diagnoses

Mild, Moderate, and Severe Mental Impairment, Cerebral Palsy, Downs Syndrome, Depression, Schizophrenia, and Bi-polar were the primary diagnoses.

Clients

The clients were between the ages of 26 and 60. They attended classrooms that were categorized by the degree of impairment. In these classrooms they are taught according to their skill level in the areas of community re-entry, ADL's, and personal safety.

Interventions

In this setting the primary interventions were bi-annual evaluations, goal and plan development, and inservicing the staff on how to implement the plan. We were available as needed to address staff and client concerns.

Sample Portfolio Page

Physical Disabilities

- **Level I Fieldwork – Tendercare Midland**
  - ☐ Case load description
    - Cerebral vascular accident, dementia, hip fracture, congestive heart failure, osteoarthritis, multiple sclerosis, parkinsons disease, wrist fracture, chronic obstructive pulmonary disorder, cerebral palsy

  - ☐ Job performance
    - Instructed geriatric population on activities of daily living, transfers, and use of adaptive equipment
    - Implemented strengthening and conditioning programs
    - Completed screening, evaluations, and discharge planning in a skilled nursing facility

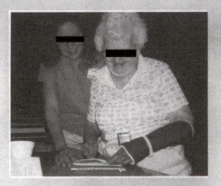

- **Level II Fieldwork – Herrick Memorial Hospital**
  - ☐ Case load description
    - Total hip arthroplasty, total knee arthroplasty, cerebral vascular accident, congestive heart failure, humerus fracture, ankle fracture, acute respiratory distress, pneumonia, acute myocardial infarction, cellulitis, compression fracture, spinal fusion, shoulder fracture, pelvic fracture, achilles tendon rupture, hepatic encephalopathy, deconditioning

  - ☐ Job Performance
    - Evaluation and treatment of clients with various diagnoses in an inpatient rehabilitative setting
    - Use of home evaluation checklists at clients residences during the discharge planning process
    - Implementation of treatment following clinical pathways and protocols in an acute care setting
    - Assisted with development of the inpatient rehabilitation evaluation form

Sample Portfolio Page

Clinical Experiences

- ## Physical Disabilities

Level I: Covenant Healthcare - Cooper Campus Acute Care
Saginaw, Michigan

This was an inpatient acute care setting. Most patients seen were orthopedic in nature, other common referring diagnoses were neurological and generalized debility. I performed chart reviews, initial evaluations and basic strengthening treatments.

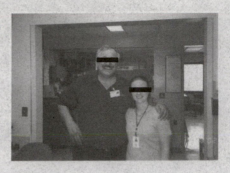

Level II: Bay Regional Medical Center - East Campus Acute Care and West Campus Outpatient Department and Rehabilitation Unit
Bay City, Michigan

First six weeks were spent in an inpatient acute care setting. I assessed and treated a nearly full caseload of patients as well as reported at team conferences on my patient's progress and rehab potential. In this setting I was exposed to many patients with orthopedic and neurologic deficits as well as those with generalized debility. For four days a week, three hours each evening, I was at the West Campus Outpatient therapy department where I was exposed to several different hand injuries; I assisted with the evaluation and treatment of the clients. I also created a splinting display board for Bay Regional Medical Center's therapist skills validation assessment day.

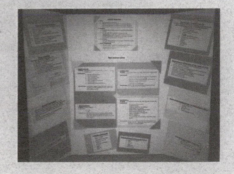

The second six weeks of my Level II fieldwork placement was spent at the inpatient rehabilitation unit. Here I assessed and treated clients in the areas of activities of daily living, functional transfers, use of adaptive equipment, home management skills, functional mobility, cognition, sensation, visual-perception, strength and endurance, and range of motion.

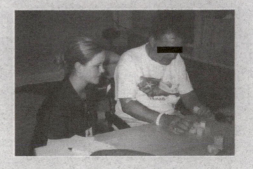

Professional Skills
10

Case Study

Name: Betty

Age: 33

Current occupation/setting: Occupational therapist in school system

Level of experience: Intermediate

Goal for portfolio: Demonstrate the need for additional occupational therapy services in her district

YOUR ABILITIES

A skill is an ability that allows a person to complete a given task. Some skills are inherent to humans, such as the ability to speak, manipulate objects, and use tools. Some skills are possessed by only a few. Although many people may try, very few can shoot a jump shot like Michael Jordan, sing like Elvis Presley, or inspire like Martin Luther King, Jr. We each possess skills inspired by our own interests and talents that identify us as uniquely capable individuals. It is these skills that the portfolio aims to highlight. What special skills do you possess? More importantly, what skills do you possess that make you the best professional for the opportunity at hand?

"Professional" is defined as the act of being engaged in a specific occupation for pay (*Webster's New World Dictionary*, 1990). Notice that the words "engaged" and "specific" are used to define professional. The use of "engaged" places emphasis on the fact that the individual has been actively involved with a set of activities. Use of the term "specific" refers to the defined skill requirements for a particular profession. The professional skills possessed by an occupational therapy professional include positive work habits along with effective interpersonal and clinical abilities or proficiencies. The practitioner is advised to carefully research constituent groups, such as the American Occupational Therapy Association (AOTA) and the National Board for Certification in Occupational Therapy (NBCOT), state regulatory bodies, and employers, to define the specific professional skills and experiences you must possess and therefore display in your portfolio in order to achieve your desired goal.

The portfolio section showcasing professional skills is your ace in the hole when it is all said and done. It lets the reader see you are capable of performing within the designated professional role. The entry-level practitioner will rely heavily on classroom activities and assignments, internship experiences, and volunteer work. Over the years, you will replace these with examples of evolving therapeutic and administrative skills and your personal style.

Occupational therapy practitioners treat clients; engage in administrative and supervisory activities; and serve as educators to clients, families, coworkers, students, and community constituents. They are also employees and coworkers. It is important that the reader formulates a clear picture of your overall strengths, capabilities, values, and goals related to professional competency. The process of collecting, selecting, organizing, and displaying is crucial to formulating that picture.

Collecting

When collecting artifacts for this section, you will want to keep pictures, brochures, print articles, samples of your professional writing (such as assessments; goals; treatment plans; discharge notes; data collection; notes from clients; supervisors and coworkers), and any other visual or print pieces that demonstrate your experiences and abilities. Be sure to eliminate any confidential and identifying references to clients, have the permission of people in your pictures or their guardians, and make sure to reference anything written by another person. Copyright laws apply to your portfolio just as they would to any other production.

Overall, the artifacts you collect to demonstrate professional skills should reflect the who, what, when, where, why, and how questions surrounding your experiences with therapeutic service.

Who Have You Worked With?

You will want those who read your portfolio to know the ages of clients you have seen. This will be particularly important if you are applying for a position in an age specific setting, such as a school system or geriatric program, or if the position requires you to be confident with clients across the lifespan. You will also want to keep track of the diagnoses and disabilities exhibited by your past clients. The reader will want to know the breadth and depth of your experience with these populations. Have you served people whose family, culture, ethnic background, race, religion, and value systems differed from your own, and were you able to effectively weave their unique needs into an appropriate treatment plan? The reader should also be able to see how you have guided, informed, and encouraged family, friends, and other significant persons in your client's life.

What Have You Done?

In discussing your ability to treat clients, it may be helpful here for you to use the occupational therapy process as a guide (Sabonis-Chafee & Hussey, 1998). This defines what occupational therapists do, and

---

Examples of What to Collect

Clinical proficiency

 ⁕ You developed a new referral process for your department to increase their client base

 ⁕ You are experienced at administering the Allen Cognitive Level Screening

 ⁕ You are trained in the use of NDT with clients

Effective interpersonal skills

 ⁕ Your annual evaluation states that one of your strengths is your ability to lead team projects effectively

 ⁕ The family of one of your clients writes a note thanking you for your help and compassion in treating their loved one

Positive work habits

 ⁕ You received an award for perfect attendance

 ⁕ You demonstrated motivation, good work ethic, and a team focus by taking on an extra project outside of your job description to assist your department in developing a new public relations campaign

---

you will be able to present your abilities and experiences related to each step.

 ⁕ Screening: Have you been involved with the development and/or implementation of screening activities?

 ⁕ Referral: With what referral agents and systems are you familiar ? Have you devised referral forms or protocols?

 ⁕ Assessment: What specific evaluations are you familiar with? How do you determine which assessment tools to use? Have you been involved in ordering and/or selecting evaluations for particular populations? Does your past experience give you expertise in assessing the needs of particular populations?

 ⁕ Problem identification: What processes do you use to determine client need?

 ⁕ Goal setting: Are you able to determine and write clear, concise, functional, measurable, and achievable goals?

 ⁕ Treatment planning: What kinds of activities do you consider appropriate for treatment? How do you determine and use available resources?

What experience do you have in developing new resources? How do you involve the client, family, coworkers, and other significant persons in this process?

✳ Treatment implementation:

What theoretical background and treatment frames of reference are you prepared to apply (i.e., nerurodevelopmental treatment (NDT), sensory integration (SI), proprioceptive neuromuscular facilitation (PNF), model of human occupation (MOHO), Cognitive Behavioral, Developmental Group Work)?

With what types of service delivery systems do you have experience (i.e., hospitals, schools, outpatient rehabilitation, community settings, day treatment)?

What experience do you have with the various service provision models and approaches (i.e., direct service, monitoring, consultation, remedial services, compensatory methods, prevention intervention strategies) (Dunn & Campbell, 1991)?

What types of treatment tools do you have experience implementing (i.e., BTE, adapted driving, computer access programs, dressing equipment, physical agent modalities, cognitive retraining software)?

What special skills have you developed (i.e., feeding, developing and fabricating assistive devices, fabricating splints, computer skills, personal counseling, behavioral management, family support and intervention)?

✳ Reassessment: How do you determine when program change or discharge is warranted?

✳ Discharge planning and follow up: What is your experience with transition, reintegration, return-to-home, and return-to-work preparation and implementation?

When Did You Become an Occupational Practitioner and How Have You Used That Time?

It is important to show continued growth in your skills over time, but it is equally important to demonstrate the quality of what you have done. Other sections of the portfolio show academic and continuing education activities, but this section allows you to personalize those experiences and show how you have applied them in practice to the benefit of clients. For example, you may choose to highlight the progressive development of skills within a particular area or specialty.

Where Have You Worked, Both in Terms of Geography and the Type of Setting?

You may also include in this section the various management and therapeutic styles within which you have worked.

Why Do You Make the Choices You Make?

Define the professional reasoning skills and value system that affects the choices you make. Each profession has developed a philosophical base made up of fundamental beliefs and values that are considered to be held by members. These evolve over time through research, trial, publication, and debate. Professional organizations such as the AOTA and state associations promote awareness and the application of these professional foundations in an effort to facilitate development of ethical, knowledgeable professionals and an educated public.

Professional decision making requires the application of critical thinking within this professional, philosophical framework. The clinical reasoning skills used by occupational practitioners in determining appropriate interventions are based in the fundamentals established by the profession as a whole.

The professional portfolio provides an avenue for demonstrating your proficiency in this critical area through examples drawn from your professional experiences. These may include artifacts, such as a list of the frames of reference you have used accompanied by photos of treatment sessions and identifying captions. You may also want to include a sample treatment plan to provide evidence of your ability to select and individualize treatment programs grounded in professional philosophy.

How Did You Organize Your Time and Manage All That Was Required of You?

This section highlights how you relate on a personal level with clients, their families, coworkers, and others. Clients must feel safe with you and trust that you are always working in their best interest. Coworkers and employers must be able to depend on you to be timely, efficient, effective, caring, and committed to the profession and the organization.

You may also want to use who, what, when, where, why, and how questions to showcase your abilities in areas of service other than client treatment. These may include administration and management, academia, research, and an ever-widening pool of career choices and directions. You may want to demonstrate how your preparation and experiences as an occupational practitioner have uniquely prepared you for a career role outside that of the typical occupational therapy arena. Your emphasis will broaden to include preferred management styles, teaching and learning theory, research interests, and other pertinent information.

Selecting

There is a potentially huge amount of information that may have been collected for this section. It is very important that you carefully consider your choices when selecting those artifacts that best meet the goals of your portfolio. The occupational therapy practitioner is qualified to work in a wide variety of settings and may be interviewing in several of these simultaneously. Do you need a selection that emphasizes your broad range of skills or do you need to focus in on a particular area of practice? You will select and emphasize different skills and experiences depending on the opportunities available. The focus of your portfolio can be altered to meet your varied needs.

Organizing

The organizing of this section may be handled in a variety of ways. For your first attempt at portfolio development, use the occupational therapy process as a guide to showcase your professional skills. This assures that you are covering all the important points by guiding the reader who may not know about occupational therapy, and educating the uninitiated on what occupational therapy practitioners do.

Collecting, Selecting, Organizing, and Displaying

Collecting
* Performance evaluations.
* Written samples of your work across the occupational therapy process including assessments, goals, treatment plans, and discharge summaries

Selecting
* The items that best meet the goals of your portfolio

Organizing
* Pair a treatment plan sample with pictures of you working with a client

Displaying
* A simplified format promoting an overall view of your abilities

---

Displaying

Displaying artifacts in the professional skills section may include lists of assessments, frames of reference, splint types, etc., as well as full documents, including reports, treatment plans, and discharge plans that are bulky. Representative pictures that encourage the reader to take a closer look may need to be placed in folders for easier management. All artifacts related to a single topic or factor should be encompassed on a single page or two facing pages to help the reader maintain focus. This is especially true in this section as the shear amount of potential information could easily become overwhelming.

Personal Application Guide

Identify your experience at each level of the occupational therapy process:

➢   Screening

➢   Referral

➢   Assessment

➢   Problem identification

➢   Goal setting

➢   Treatment planning

➢   Treatment implementation

➢   Re-assessment

➢   Discharge planning and follow up

Selecting Guide

Professional Skills

In the circles, write down each achievement, skill, and/or characteristic that you want showcased in your portfolio. Next to the circles, write which artifacts you will use to demonstrate the achievement. You may not have an artifact for each achievement, so you may choose to use a list of brief description instead.

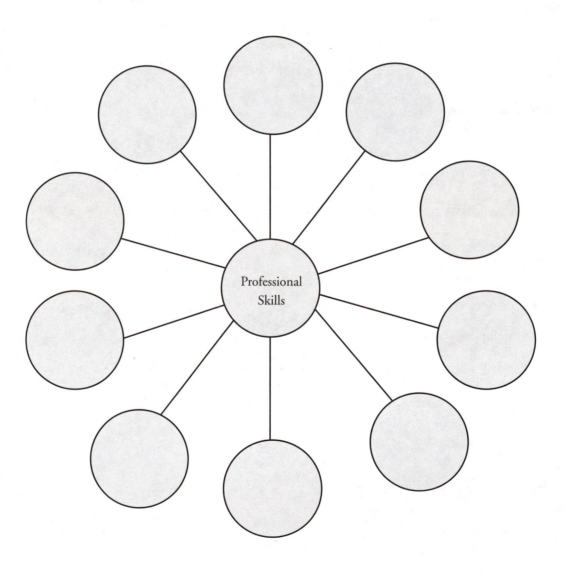

Selecting Guide

Professional Skills: Sample Response

I am going to demonstrate how I use my skills as an OT to achieve these by using a case study for each one with pictures; a chart of other students that I have helped in each area; and how improvements in each area impact other areas of school performance for the student, their classmates, the classroom environment, and for teachers.

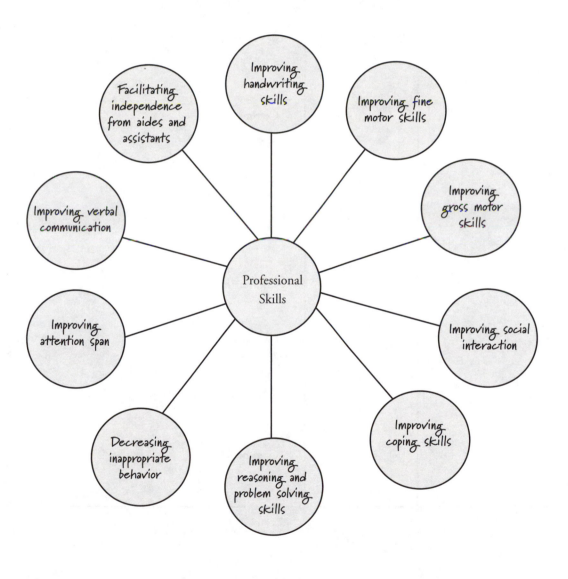

Self Assessment

Professional Skills

After reviewing your portfolio, grade each of the categories below with a score between 1 and 5 (1 = poor, 3 = good, 5 = excellent). Feel free to make any comments you feel necessary.

Neatness	1 2 3 4 5	Comments:
Organization	1 2 3 4 5	Comments:
Completeness	1 2 3 4 5	Comments:
Content	1 2 3 4 5	Comments:
Relevancy	1 2 3 4 5	Comments:
Flow	1 2 3 4 5	Comments:
Consistency	1 2 3 4 5	Comments:
Visual appearance	1 2 3 4 5	Comments:
Representative of you	1 2 3 4 5	Comments:
Appropriate amount of info	1 2 3 4 5	Comments:

Peer Evaluation

Professional Skills

After reviewing your peer's portfolio, grade each of the categories below with a score between 1 and 5 (1 = poor, 3 = good, 5 = excellent). Feel free to make any comments you feel necessary.

Neatness	1 2 3 4 5	Comments:
Organization	1 2 3 4 5	Comments:
Completeness	1 2 3 4 5	Comments:
Content	1 2 3 4 5	Comments:
Relevancy	1 2 3 4 5	Comments:
Flow	1 2 3 4 5	Comments:
Consistency	1 2 3 4 5	Comments:
Visual appearance	1 2 3 4 5	Comments:
Representative of you	1 2 3 4 5	Comments:
Appropriate amount of info	1 2 3 4 5	Comments:

Peer evaluator's name:

Date:

Sample Portfolio Page

Adaptive Toys and Switches

Creating a switch operated toy by hard wiring the battery compartment to a switch compatible jack was one way that I learned to adapt a toy. Another way was to create a battery adapter or "pigtail" (pictured right) which allows for any battery operated toy to be connected to a switch.

Adaptive Equipment

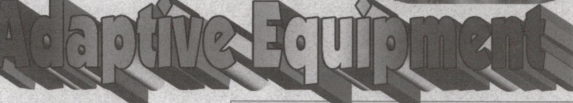

I developed an adaptive device to allow individuals without adequate grip strength and/or manipulation skills to shave.

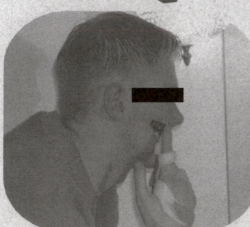

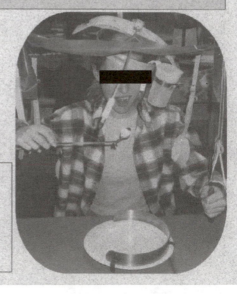

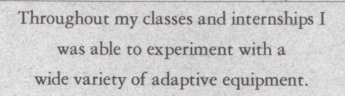

Throughout my classes and internships I was able to experiment with a wide variety of adaptive equipment.

Sample Portfolio Page

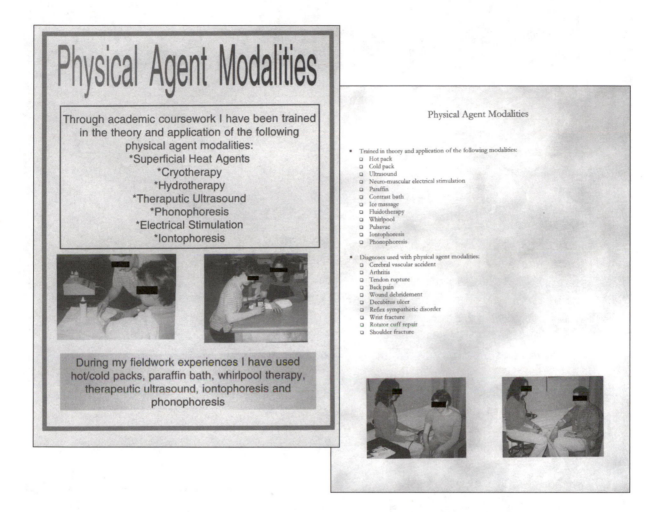

Here are two samples of how to display your abilities and experiences with physical agent modalities. Notice how the pictures demonstrating the occupational therapy practitioner utilizing various physical agents are used in conjunction with lists to give extra visual appeal and interest. What experience do you have with each physical agent?

— **Sample Portfolio Page** —

Screening and Assessment

*Goniometry, Dynamometer
*Edema Assessment: (Tape and Displacement Methods)
*GreenLeaf Medical, Eval Solo System
*Manual Muscle Testing
*Valpar Work Sampling
*Self-Care Observation
*Mini-Mental State Evaluation
*Motor Free Visual Perceptual Test-Revised (MVPT-R)
*Developmental Test of Visual Motor Integration(VMI)
*Infant/Toddler Symptom Checklist
*Test of Pictures/Letters/Numbers/Spatial Orientation & Sequencing Skills
*Allen Cognitive Level Screen (ACL)
*Lerner Magazine Collage
*Comprehensive Occupational Therapy Evaluation (COTE)
*Role Checklist
*Interest Checklist
*Geriatric Depression Scale
*Wide Range Assessment of Visual Motor Abilities
*Peabody Developmental Motor Scales
*VMI
*Developmental Checklists

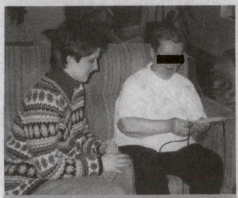

Administering the Allen Cognitive Level Screen on my Level One Fieldwork at PineCrest Farms in Midland, Michigan.

TEAM EVALUATION

Through professional employment at Covenant Healthcare and Fieldwork experience at Bay-Arenac ISD I have used several approaches to team evaluation and treatment planning.
For example:
   *Infant and toddler evaluations and IEP formulation during fieldwork.
   *At Covenant we use a multidisciplinary approach to both assessment and treatment planning.
(Please Refer to Documentation Folder)

Professional Employment

RehabCare at Covenant HealthCare
510 N. Michigan Ave.
Saginaw, Michigan

Supervisor: Diane Glasgow OTR

Employment Dates: March 5, 2001 to present

Position: Occupational Therapist (OTR)

Employment Status: Full Time

RehabCare Group

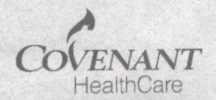

This Program is an Inpatient Rehabilitation Program. I am pictured at Right with a patient and therapist at our rehab carnival during National Rehabilitation Week.

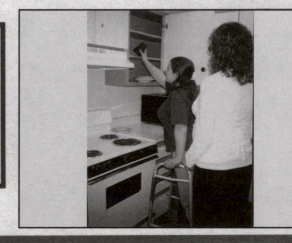

Sample Portfolio Page

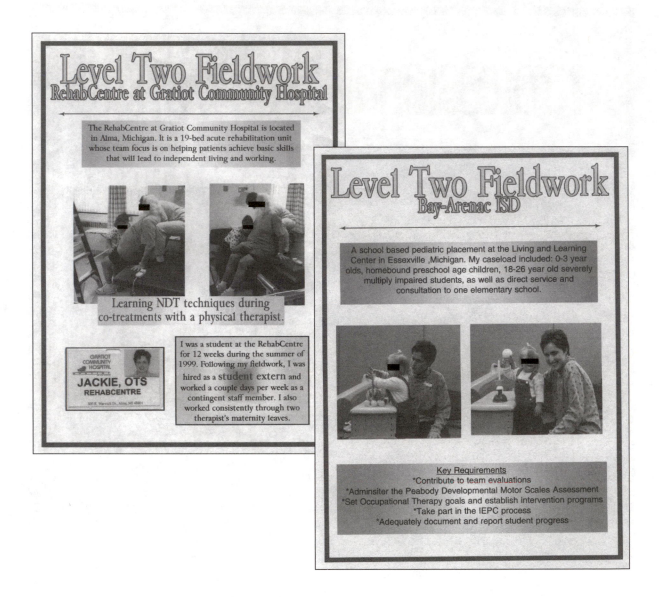

This is one example of how the same experience can be used in two different sections. Here, the occupational therapy student uses her fieldwork experiences in the professional skills section instead of in the professional development section. Remember, this is your portfolio, so use your experiences and artifacts in a way that makes sense to you and best represents your abilities.

Sample Portfolio Page

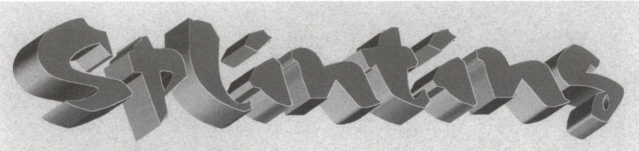

During three days of interactive workshops I learned the fundamentals of static and dynamic splinting.

The topics covered included:

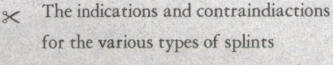
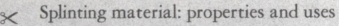
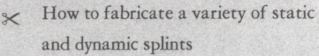
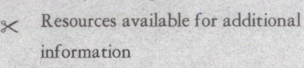

✂ The indications and contraindiactions for the various types of splints

✂ Splinting material: properties and uses

✂ How to fabricate a variety of static and dynamic splints

✂ Resources available for additional information

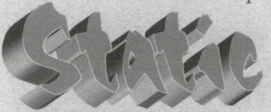

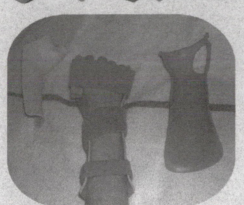

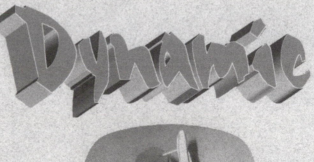

I fabricated five different splints using five different materials.

↑ Pictured above are three of the four static splints (thumb spica splint, functional hand splint, and wrist cock-up splint).

⇒ To the right is the dynamic splint that I fabricated.

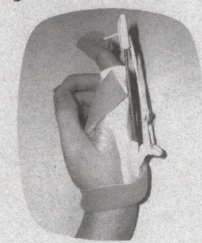

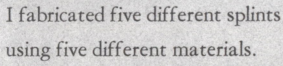

Sample Portfolio Page

Professional Skill Development

Date	Skill	Training Received

Professional Presentations and Publications 11

Case Study

Name: Pam

Age: 42

Current occupation/setting: OTA in work hardening/return-to work-program

Level of experience: Experienced

Goal for portfolio: Make the move to private practice in same setting

---

Case Study

Name: Bob

Age: 37

Current occupation/setting: Occupational therapy—community mental health/home care

Level of experience: Experienced

Goal for portfolio: Recertification

SHARING INFORMATION

An important professional obligation is the sharing of information related to areas of particular skill and interest. That is one way in which the profession as a whole develops. Occupational therapy practitioners who engage in these activities demonstrate an advanced level of commitment to the profession and their own growth. The intermediate and advanced practitioner may have multiple examples, while the student and entry-level practitioner may have engaged in very few or even none of these experiences. If the latter is the case, you will want the reviewer to know that you value the activity and have plans for the future. You may want to include areas of interest for future presentations and publications or, at the very least, demonstrate how you are preparing to engage in this activity in the future. Academic programs may consider this a push to provide opportunities and support for their students to engage in public speaking and publication outside the educational setting.

Collecting

Collecting is much the same for your own presentations as it is for those of others you attend. A charting system will be the most efficient method, along with a copy of the content presented and to whom you presented. Pictures are also helpful. You will want to keep any feedback you receive from participants regarding your skills as a presenter and the usefulness of the content.

Publications may be managed through use of a chronological bibliography system. Each citation should be accompanied by a very brief summary of the content. Short print articles may be maintained in their entirety. Include any critical review or feedback related to the publication.

Selection

Selection may mean including all items on your chart and/or bibliography or making judicious selections around a particular topic or practice area. Carefully select only a very limited number of accompanying artifacts.

Organizing

Material in these two sections will be self-organizing and often very brief. This can act as an encouragement to share more of yourself.

Collecting, Selecting, Organizing, and Displaying

Collecting
* Chart presentation dates and summarize content
* Chart publications and dates

Selecting
* A summary of all items in list or chart form

Organizing
* Factual information
* Supportive pictures and documents

Displaying
* A simplified format promoting an overall view of accomplishments

Displaying

The display of these materials should make it very clear that you are the originator and author of the content. Keep the pages clean and clear. Maintain continuity with the overall style of your portfolio, but focus on the material. The chart provided here will get you started on the collection process and will adequately maintain a lifetime log of your activities.

Selecting Guide

Professional Presentations

In the circles, write down each achievement, skill, and/or characteristic that you want showcased in your portfolio. Next to the circles, write which artifacts you will use to demonstrate the achievement. You may not have an artifact for each achievement, so you may choose to use a list of brief description instead.

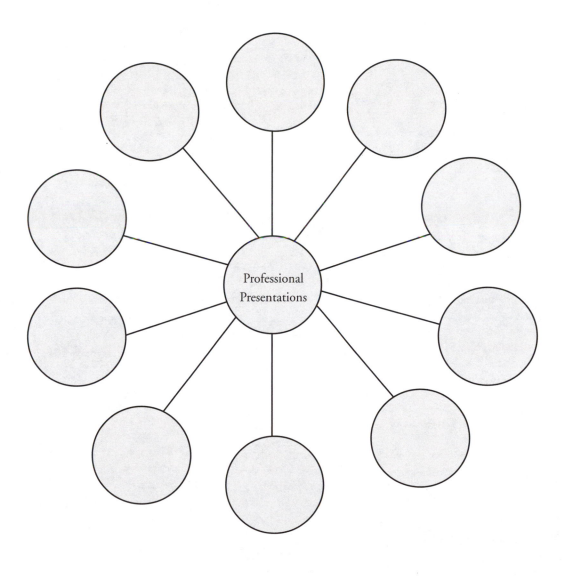

Professional Presentations

Selecting Guide

Professional Presentations: Sample Response

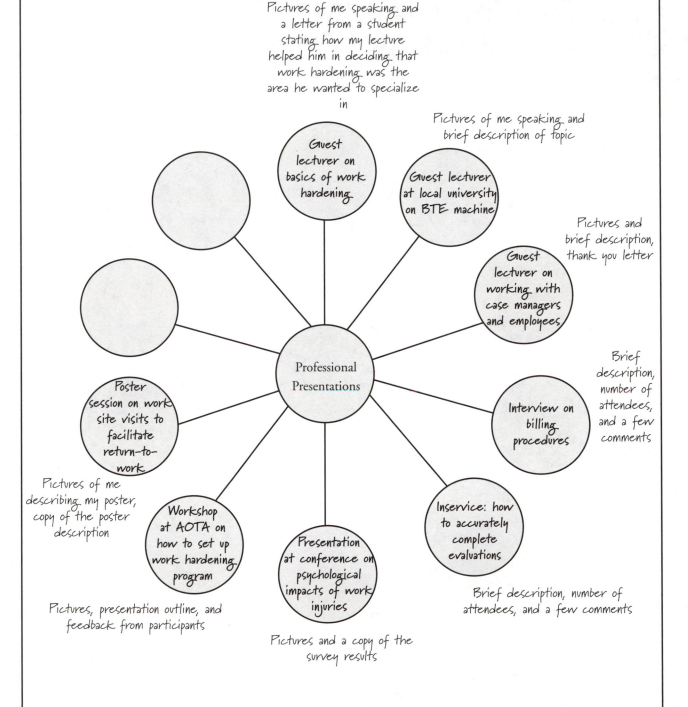

Pictures of me speaking and a letter from a student stating how my lecture helped him in deciding that work hardening was the area he wanted to specialize in

Guest lecturer on basics of work hardening

Pictures of me speaking and brief description of topic

Guest lecturer at local university on BTE machine

Pictures and brief description, thank you letter

Guest lecturer on working with case managers and employees

Professional Presentations

Brief description, number of attendees, and a few comments

Interview on billing procedures

Poster session on work site visits to facilitate return-to-work

Pictures of me describing my poster, copy of the poster description

Workshop at AOTA on how to set up work hardening program

Presentation at conference on psychological impacts of work injuries

Inservice: how to accurately complete evaluations

Brief description, number of attendees, and a few comments

Pictures, presentation outline, and feedback from participants

Pictures and a copy of the survey results

Selecting Guide

Professional Publications

In the circles, write down each achievement, skill, and/or characteristic that you want showcased in your portfolio. Next to the circles, write which artifacts you will use to demonstrate the achievement. You may not have an artifact for each achievement, so you may choose to use a list of brief description instead.

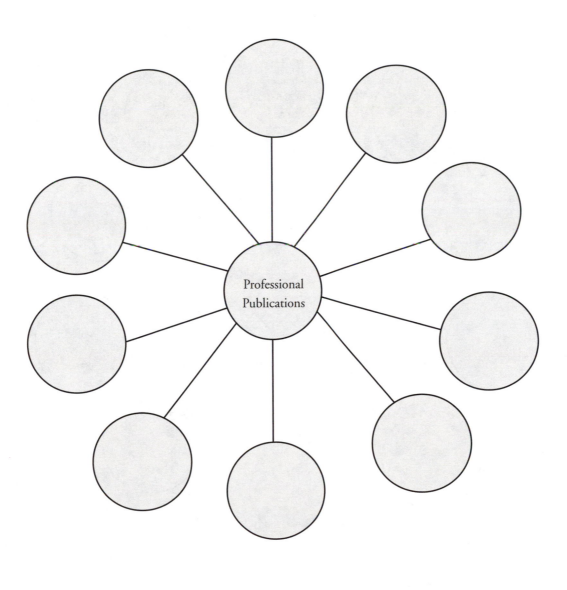

Selecting Guide

Professional Publications: Sample Response

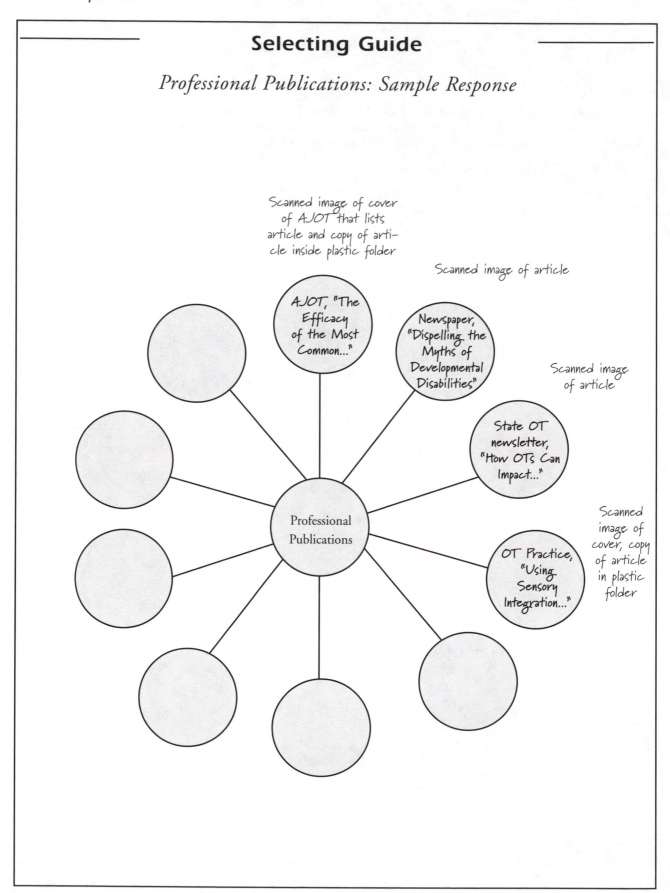

Scanned image of cover of AJOT that lists article and copy of article inside plastic folder

Scanned image of article

Scanned image of article

Scanned image of cover, copy of article in plastic folder

AJOT, "The Efficacy of the Most Common..."

Newspaper, "Dispelling the Myths of Developmental Disabilities"

State OT newsletter, "How OTs Can Impact..."

OT Practice, "Using Sensory Integration..."

Professional Publications

Self Assessment

Professional Publications and Presentations

After reviewing your portfolio, grade each of the categories below with a score between 1 and 5 (1 = poor, 3 = good, 5 = excellent). Feel free to make any comments you feel necessary.

Neatness	1 2 3 4 5	Comments:
Organization	1 2 3 4 5	Comments:
Completeness	1 2 3 4 5	Comments:
Content	1 2 3 4 5	Comments:
Relevancy	1 2 3 4 5	Comments:
Flow	1 2 3 4 5	Comments:
Consistency	1 2 3 4 5	Comments:
Visual appearance	1 2 3 4 5	Comments:
Representative of you	1 2 3 4 5	Comments:
Appropriate amount of info	1 2 3 4 5	Comments:

Peer Evaluation

Professional Presentations and Publications

After reviewing your peer's portfolio, grade each of the categories below with a score between 1 and 5 (1 = poor, 3 = good, 5 = excellent). Feel free to make any comments you feel necessary.

Neatness	1 2 3 4 5	Comments:
Organization	1 2 3 4 5	Comments:
Completeness	1 2 3 4 5	Comments:
Content	1 2 3 4 5	Comments:
Relevancy	1 2 3 4 5	Comments:
Flow	1 2 3 4 5	Comments:
Consistency	1 2 3 4 5	Comments:
Visual appearance	1 2 3 4 5	Comments:
Representative of you	1 2 3 4 5	Comments:
Appropriate amount of info	1 2 3 4 5	Comments:

Peer evaluator's name:

Date:

— Sample Portfolio Page —

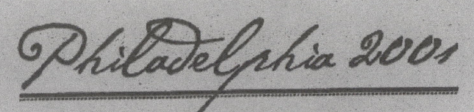

Philadelphia 2001

AOTA's Annual Conference & Exposition
Thursday, April 19–Sunday, April 22

Are OT's using Physical Agents? A Survey of Michigan OT's

~This was a presentation and discussion regarding a research project completed during my senior year at SVSU. I presented the project with three other OT Graduates who also took part in completing the research.

The Professional Portfolio: Development and Use Throughout Professional Life

~This presentation was a short course aimed at educating OT's regarding the use of portfolios. Our goal was to teach participants how the portfolio can support the therapist and the field of OT by articulating skills and accomplishments and guiding professional development. This presentation was met with such overwhelming interest, that we are currently working on a published version.

Sample Portfolio Page

Conference Presentations
Michigan Occupational Therapy Association
1999 Fall Conference

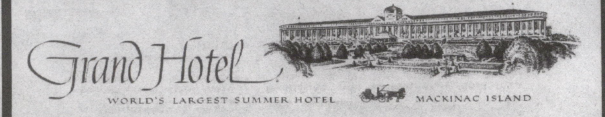

Grand Hotel
WORLD'S LARGEST SUMMER HOTEL   MACKINAC ISLAND

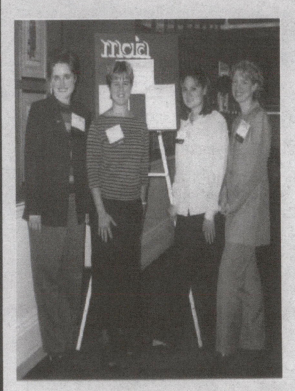

Proprioceptive
Neuromuscular Facilitation:
The Basics for Use in
Occupational Therapy

This presentation began as
a class project. With the
encouragement and
assistance of our professor
we submitted the project to
the MOTA call for papers.

— **Sample Portfolio Page** —

Inservices and Workshops I Have Given:

1. Transfer Workshops
   *I have taken part in 3 transfer training workshops for nursing
   students at SVSU.

2. Proprioceptive Neuromuscular Facilitation:
   *Diagonal Inservice on my Level One at Covenant Healthcare
   *PNF Techniques Inservice on my Level Two Fieldwork in Alma
   *MOTA Conference Workshop

3. Finding Room for Spiritualism in Occupational Therapy
   *Class Presentation
   *MOTA, Student Educational Symposium

4. Alzheimer's Disease and Home Safety
   *During my level two fieldwork in Alma, I presented about home
   safety for individuals with dementia at a caregiver support group
   meeting.

Class Presentations/Inservices Given

1. Systemic Lupus Erythematosus
2. Developmental Dyspraxia
3. An In Depth Look at the American Occupational Therapy Assn.
4. Therapeutic Use of Humor
5. Manual Therapy Treatment Techniques
6. Integrative Group Therapy: A Sensory Integration Group

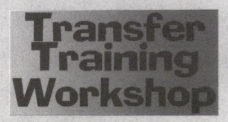

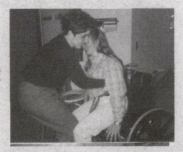

Sample Portfolio Page

Professional Publications (cont.)

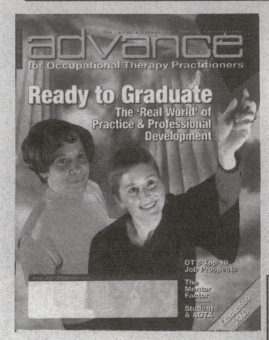

What kind of help has your mentor been to you?
"Mrs. Nagayda was my first OT teacher for Intro to OT, and that was actually before I entered the program. That was probably the first point where I knew I had someone I could go to and talk to, which was very helpful because I could ask her questions [about the program]. Mrs. Nagayda's field of practice is in pediatrics—she has 15 years of experience—so she has a lot of great examples from her own practice. I am interested in pediatrics, so I see Mrs. Nagayda as a resource in the future if that is what I pursue. [The professors] are always getting calls back from graduates of the program asking for advice and new treatment ideas, so I know that that door is always open and that I can always call."

Jennifer Sequin
Saginaw Valley State University, Michigan
SVS Student OT Association President
Anticipated Graduation Date: Aug. 14, 2003
Mentor: Janet Nagayda, BS, MS, associate professor of SVS OT dept.

A fellow classmate and I were interviewed for the March 24ᵗʰ Issue of "Advance for Occupational Therapy Practitioners." The article discussed the importance of having a mentor in one's personal and professional life.

Sample Portfolio Page

Professional Publications (cont.)

OT Perspectives

October 20, 2002   Volume 1, Issue 1, Fall 2002

Presidents Address- 2002-2003 Is Off To A Rip-Roaring Start!

Jennifer Sequin, SOTA President

As we head into the eighth week of the Fall 2002 semester it is almost inconceivable to think that the semester is already halfway through! Amongst demanding class assignments, projects, report deadlines, and exams, SOTA has still managed to partake in some very worthwhile events on and around campus.

To start the semester off, several OT students conducted a training workshop on proper patient transferring techniques for the first semester nursing students. Soon after, SOTA elections were held for the Junior class. Next came the Junior/Senior pizza party. More recently, many members of the Senior OT class participated in the annual Homecoming festivities which included making a spirit banner, constructing a float, and participating in the parade; not to mention nominating one of our very own for homecoming queen.

On top of classes, and the previously mentioned events, students have been hard at work preparing for the OT conference to be held on November 13. Committees have been formed to cover the many duties including scheduling speakers, creating brochures, contacting area practitioners, collecting donations for a raffle, promotion of the event, and much more. We are also currently in the middle of a fundraising project.

All of the activities already completed and those yet to come are preformed with the intent with promoting Occupational Therapy within our own program, on campus, and in the community— and also to expand and enhance each students interpretation and understanding of OT. I look forward to future participation in such events including working with the community, charitable organizations, Disability Awareness Week, and a holiday party for all OT students.

In *October of 2002* I wrote the President's Address article for the *OT Perspectives* newsletter. As President of Student Occupational Therapy Association (SOTA) at SVSU, at this time I summarized the fall 2002 semester as well as highlighted the activities SOTA had been involved with.

Service

12

Case Study

Name: Mary

Age: 35

Current occupation/setting: Occupational therapy student

Level of experience: Student

Goal for portfolio: Looking for employment in pediatric rehabilitation setting

HELPING OTHERS AND DEVELOPING SKILLS

The artifacts in this section reflect activities you have engaged in without regard to remuneration. They have been undertaken to support your profession and humanity. Service activities include serving on local, state, or national professional boards or activity groups; engaging in public relations activities; or other activities that promote the growth and development of the profession. When we endeavor to improve our communities and the human condition, we are enacting our beliefs about the value of people and the role of society in supporting the quality of human life. These activities may include things like volunteering to work within agencies such as Habitat for Humanity, Special Olympics, the Red Cross, and Big Brothers/Big Sisters. We may also lend our energies to various political activities, such as a local school board or government office. During all of these activities, we are helping our neighbors and developing skills and contacts that will benefit our clients and profession.

Collecting

Collecting artifacts for this area may involve letters of thanks, commendations, newspaper articles, pictures, and a wide variety of other items. It may be a challenge to find visual representations for all of the many activities in which you engage. Keep a log of all of your activities so you can at least report a date and description of what you did.

Selecting

The selection of items for this section requires a careful evaluation of each item to assure that you only use those that are really necessary. Check with your overall goals of the portfolio and select only those artifacts that really fit with the purpose.

Organizing

Organizing the artifacts for this section can usually be done with a little more flair than may be apparent in other sections. Your personality may show through more here because the service activities you chose to engage in are a reflection of your values and special interests.

Displaying

Try to let the display style reflect your personal style, as well as fit with the kinds of activities you have chosen. While you may have some type of list to chronicle the events as they occur, the display will have more impact if you use pictures and other artifacts to highlight your participation and the results of your efforts. This section may have more of a scrapbook feel.

Collecting, Selecting, Organizing, and Displaying

Collecting
*   Letters of thanks
*   Newspaper articles
*   Pictures
*   Certificates of participation
*   Keep a log documenting service activities

Selecting
*   Activities that support the overall goal/purpose of your portfolio
*   Artifacts that reflect your values and goals

Organizing
*   Let your personality show through

Displaying
*   Use pictures for greater impact
*   Make sure you are showing off the results of your efforts

Selecting Guide

Service

In the circles, write down each achievement, skill, and/or characteristic that you want showcased in your portfolio. Next to the circles, write which artifacts you will use to demonstrate the achievement. You may not have an artifact for each achievement, so you may choose to use a list of brief description instead.

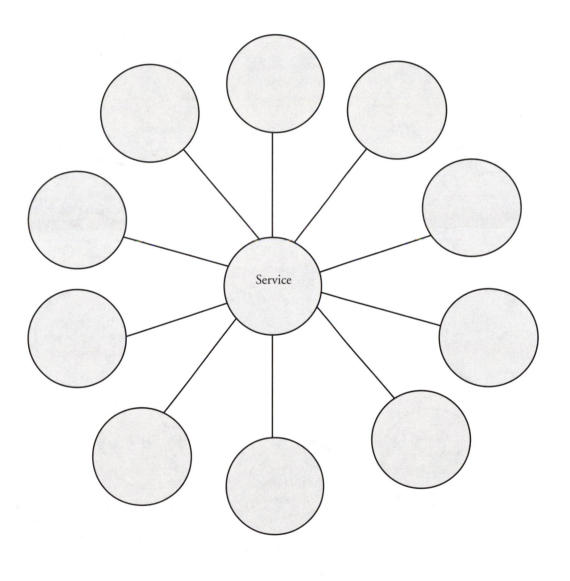

Selecting Guide

Service: Sample Response

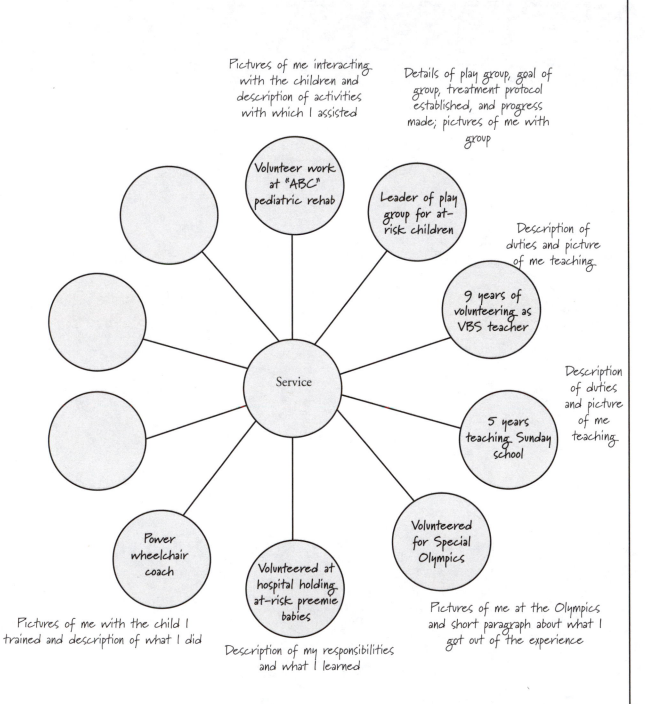

Pictures of me interacting with the children and description of activities with which I assisted

Details of play group, goal of group, treatment protocol established, and progress made; pictures of me with group

Volunteer work at "ABC" pediatric rehab

Leader of play group for at-risk children

Description of duties and picture of me teaching

9 years of volunteering as VBS teacher

Service

5 years teaching Sunday school

Description of duties and picture of me teaching

Volunteered for Special Olympics

Power wheelchair coach

Volunteered at hospital holding at-risk preemie babies

Pictures of me with the child I trained and description of what I did

Description of my responsibilities and what I learned

Pictures of me at the Olympics and short paragraph about what I got out of the experience

Self Assessment

Service

After reviewing your portfolio, grade each of the categories below with a score between 1 and 5 (1 = poor, 3 = good, 5 = excellent). Feel free to make any comments you feel necessary.

Neatness	1 2 3 4 5	Comments:
Organization	1 2 3 4 5	Comments:
Completeness	1 2 3 4 5	Comments:
Content	1 2 3 4 5	Comments:
Relevancy	1 2 3 4 5	Comments:
Flow	1 2 3 4 5	Comments:
Consistency	1 2 3 4 5	Comments:
Visual appearance	1 2 3 4 5	Comments:
Representative of you	1 2 3 4 5	Comments:
Appropriate amount of info	1 2 3 4 5	Comments:

Peer Evaluation

Service

After reviewing your peer's portfolio, grade each of the categories below with a score between 1 and 5 (1 = poor, 3 = good, 5 = excellent). Feel free to make any comments you feel necessary.

Neatness	1 2 3 4 5	Comments:
Organization	1 2 3 4 5	Comments:
Completeness	1 2 3 4 5	Comments:
Content	1 2 3 4 5	Comments:
Relevancy	1 2 3 4 5	Comments:
Flow	1 2 3 4 5	Comments:
Consistency	1 2 3 4 5	Comments:
Visual appearance	1 2 3 4 5	Comments:
Representative of you	1 2 3 4 5	Comments:
Appropriate amount of info	1 2 3 4 5	Comments:

Peer evaluator's name:

Date:

── Sample Portfolio Page ──

Professional Service

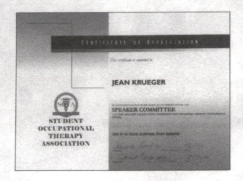

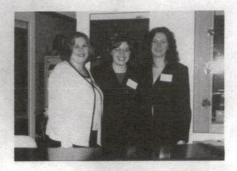

March 2002
- Served as Head of the Speaker Committee at the Saginaw Valley State University Occupational Therapy Conference

2001 – 2002
- Served as Public Relations Officer for the Student Occupational Therapy Association at Saginaw Valley State University

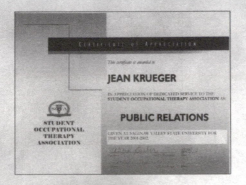

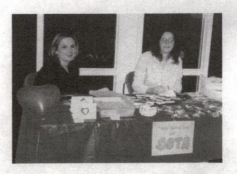

Sample Portfolio Page

Community Service

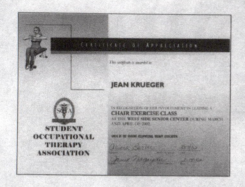

March 2002 – April 2002
- Assisted in leading a chair exercise program at the West Side Senior Center through the Saginaw County Commission on Aging

November 2000
- East Side Soup Kitchen – Canned food drive

December 2000
- Families in need – Holiday gift donations through Salvation Army

January 2001
- City Rescue Mission – Book drive

December 2001
- Families in need – Holiday gift giving through United Way

November 2000
- Attended a tour and luncheon at the City Rescue Mission in Saginaw, Michigan

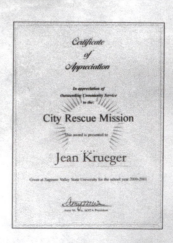

Sample Portfolio Page

Community Service

1st Annual Great Lakes Wheelchair Rugby Tournament
October 19, 2002 - SVSU

Three fellow classmates and I volunteered to keep score, monitor timeouts and penalties, and assist the disabled rugby players in any way they needed.

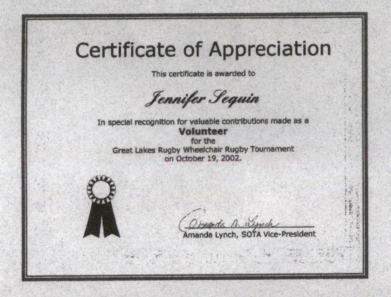

Certificate of Appreciation

This certificate is awarded to

Jennifer Seguin

In special recognition for valuable contributions made as a
Volunteer
for the
Great Lakes Rugby Wheelchair Rugby Tournament
on October 19, 2002.

Amanda Lynch, SOTA Vice-President

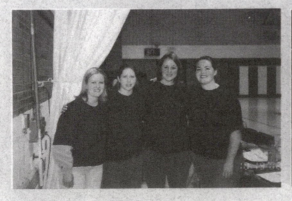
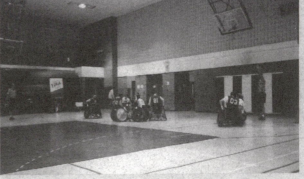

Wheelchair Basketball
at the Millet Center

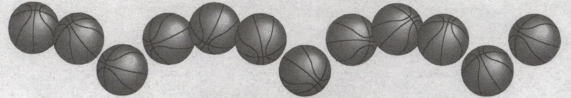

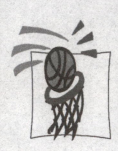

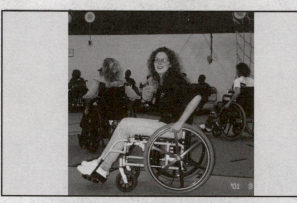

Each year, students in the occupational therapy program make several trips to the Millet Learning Center in Bridgeport, Michigan. One of our favorite trips is when the children challenge us to a game of wheelchair basketball!

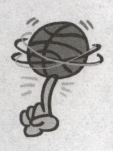

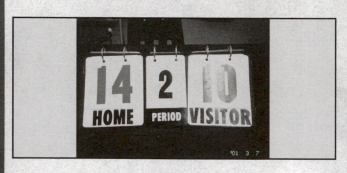

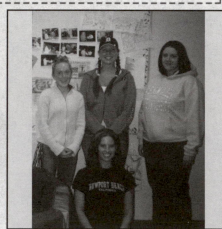

Expressions of Support

13

Case Study

Name: Brad

Age: 22

Current occupation/setting: OTA in outpatient rehabilitation facility

Level of experience: Entry-level

Goal for portfolio: Seeking full-time employment

Collecting, Selecting, Organizing, and Displaying

Collecting
* Letters of reference
* Memos
* Thank you notes, letters, and drawings

Selecting
* Items related to the portfolio purpose
* Artifacts demonstrating support from co-workers, clients, families, and community sources

Organizing
* Combine the support items, pictures, or drawings

Displaying
* Formal items, a formal display
* Informal items, an informal display
* May be displayed separately from one another or they can be interspersed

DIFFERENT FORMS OF EXPRESSION

There are many times when clients, coworkers, and others will let you know you have made a difference in their lives, done something above and beyond what was expected, or are appreciated. At times, these are very formal, as with letters of recommendation. They can take many other forms like a picture a child draws for you, a letter from a client and her family, or a thank you note from a coworker. All of these help fill out the picture of who you are.

Collecting

Collecting these items requires care because people often don't value them as they should. Save all of these, even memos, as they come to you. Even if they don't make their way into your portfolio, they are good to look at from time to time. They will remind you that even the small things you do are important and can have repercussions you never expected.

Selecting

Select items for your portfolio that best reflect those characteristics you are hoping to bring to the reviewer's attention.

Organization and Display

The organization and display artifacts here will be determined by the type of item. Formal letters and commendations will be displayed formally. Informal and personal pieces can be displayed in a way that best suits their nature. If including letters and notes, it is a good idea to use a highlighter to mark information to which you want to draw attention.

Selecting Guide

Expressions of Support

In the circles, write down each achievement, skill, and/or characteristic that you want showcased in your portfolio. Next to the circles, write which artifacts you will use to demonstrate the achievement. You may not have an artifact for each achievement, so you may choose to use a list of brief description instead.

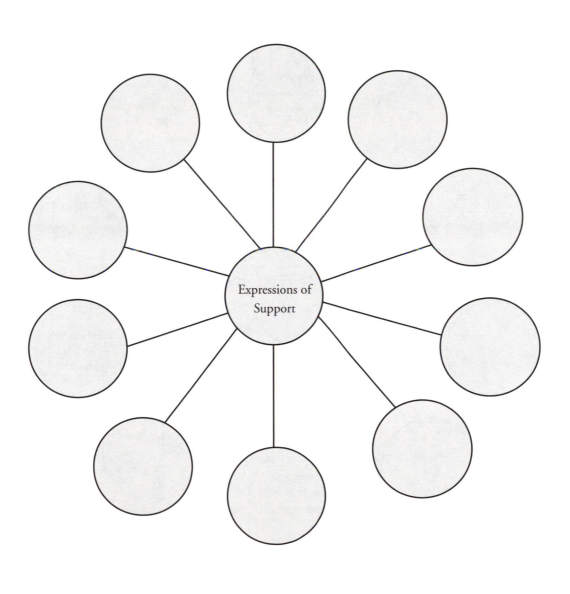

Expressions of Support

Selecting Guide

Expressions of Support: Sample Response

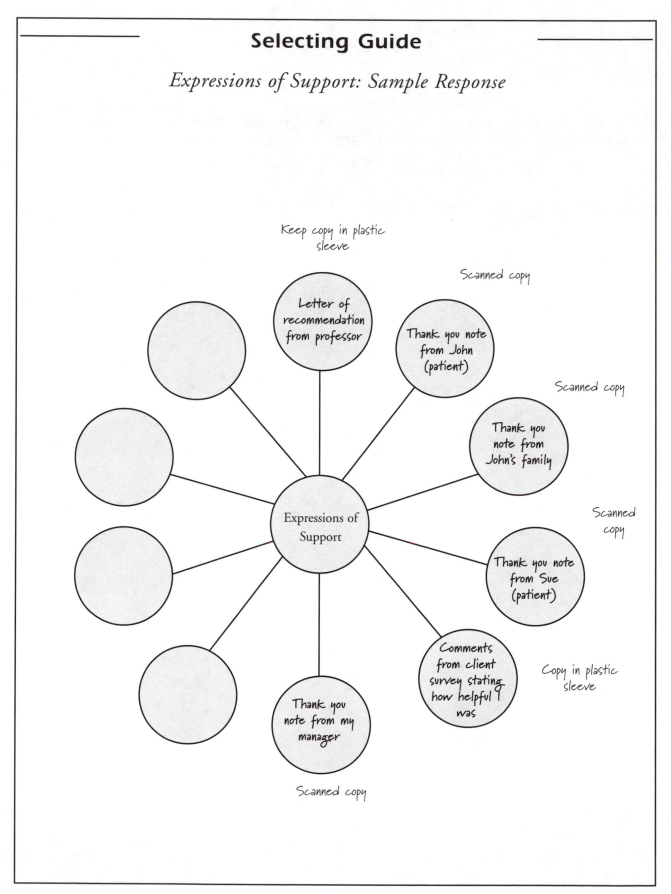

Self Assessment

Expressions of Support

After reviewing your portfolio, grade each of the categories below with a score between 1 and 5 (1 = poor, 3 = good, 5 = excellent). Feel free to make any comments you feel necessary.

Neatness	1 2 3 4 5	Comments:
Organization	1 2 3 4 5	Comments:
Completeness	1 2 3 4 5	Comments:
Content	1 2 3 4 5	Comments:
Relevancy	1 2 3 4 5	Comments:
Flow	1 2 3 4 5	Comments:
Consistency	1 2 3 4 5	Comments:
Visual appearance	1 2 3 4 5	Comments:
Representative of you	1 2 3 4 5	Comments:
Appropriate amount of info	1 2 3 4 5	Comments:

Peer Evaluation

Expressions of Support

After reviewing your peer's portfolio, grade each of the categories below with a score between 1 and 5 (1 = poor, 3 = good, 5 = excellent). Feel free to make any comments you feel necessary.

Neatness	1 2 3 4 5	Comments:
Organization	1 2 3 4 5	Comments:
Completeness	1 2 3 4 5	Comments:
Content	1 2 3 4 5	Comments:
Relevancy	1 2 3 4 5	Comments:
Flow	1 2 3 4 5	Comments:
Consistency	1 2 3 4 5	Comments:
Visual appearance	1 2 3 4 5	Comments:
Representative of you	1 2 3 4 5	Comments:
Appropriate amount of info	1 2 3 4 5	Comments:

Peer evaluator's name:

Date:

Sample Portfolio Page

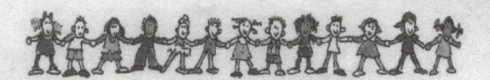

9680 Janes Rd
Saginaw, MI 4860
April 4, 2001

RE: Letter of reference for Sarah Schindehette

In July of 1999 my husband, Norm suffered a massive CVA. He had therapy at Covenant South Campus and also outpatient therapy till we met the limit that the insurance would cover. Unable to continue the therapy as an outpatient we were advised to contact the local universities and inquire for a student to work with my husband.

We were apprehensive, but felt that it was vital that we at least try. When Sarah called to inquire about the position, it was an answer to our prayers. We knew Sarah through our church, and also know her parents.

Sarah met with us and together we evaluated the situation and decided that we would have Sarah work with Norm 3 times a week. It was the best decision we made.

Even though Norm and I wanted to continue to do therapy on our own, we were at odds and ended up more frustrated than productive. Sarah was able with authority, yet sweetness and compassion guide both Norm and myself in the proper way to regain strength in his left side. She has been efficient and conscientious, motivating Norm to continue to stretch for the next level of recovery. Sarah is always watchful for ways to encourage Norm, knowing when he needed to be pushed a little and knowing when he simply needs TLC

She also works well with the physical therapist. If schedules allow, they work once a week as a team with Norm. Sarah is cooperative and supportive and the two work with respect for each other.

We have spoken with Sarah of her ambition to work with young children. We have also seen her abilities to relate with children. Our granddaughter who was 9 months old when Sarah started coming is very comfortable with Sarah. She has that touch that enables children to trust her.

Sarah's influence and knowledge, her skills and personality have been vital in Norm's recovery. The progress he has made has been outstanding. We hope to have Sarah's continued involvement with Norm's recovery. We trust her integrity and loyalty and know that if circumstances warrant changes, we would be thankful for the time she has spent with us and wish her God's blessings and with confidence know that she will do the best she can in her vocation.

Respectfully,

Catherine M. Reinert

Catherine M. Reinert

Sample Portfolio Page

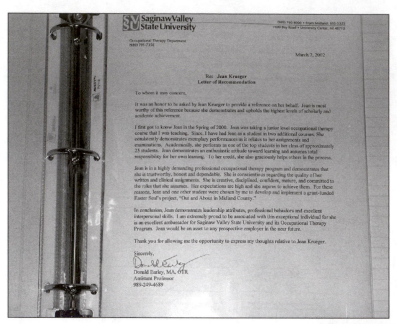

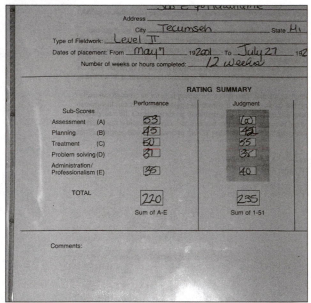

You can use letters of reference and evaluations, such as the American Occupational Therapy Association fieldwork evaluation, to demonstrate how others support you in your work and perceive your abilities.

Sample Portfolio Page

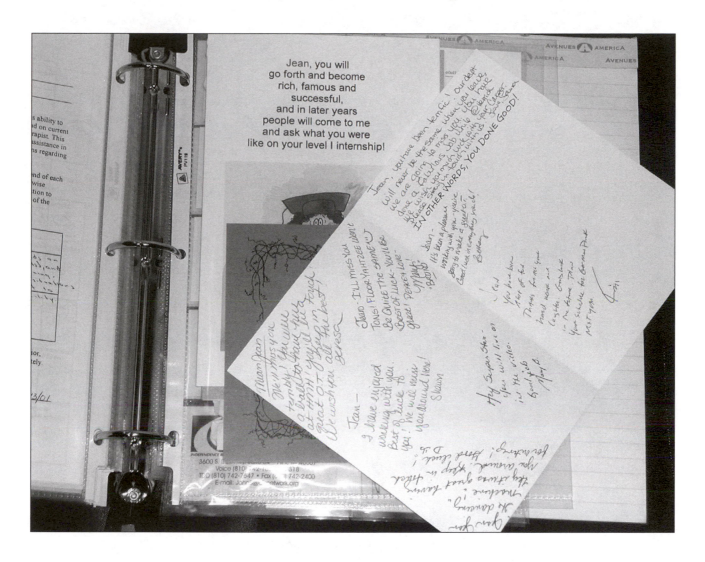

Cards; thank you notes; and supportive notes from supervisors, clients, families, and peers can be displayed in a clear plastic sleeve.

Personal 14

Case Study

Name: Samantha

Age: 28

Current occupation/setting: Occupational therapy student

Level of experience: Student

Goal for portfolio: Applying for an internship at an inpatient psychiatric facility

Collecting, Selecting, Organizing, and Displaying

Collecting
* Artifacts regarding hobbies, clubs, and non-professional membership
* Family photos

Selecting
* Artifacts that are important to you
* Something important you feel a potential employer should know about you

Organizing
* Show how your personal life enhances your professional life

Displaying
* Let your personal style shine
* This section really reflects you

This section is optional and should only be included if there are aspects of your personal life that you want others to consider. If something is sufficiently important in your life and you feel a potential employer or other reader should know about it, this is where the information is incorporated. You may wish to emphasize your family life or an activity that is particularly important to you. It may also be helpful to identify how one or more aspects of the activities enhances your professional life.

Selecting Guide

Personal

In the circles, write down each achievement, skill, and/or characteristic that you want showcased in your portfolio. Next to the circles, write which artifacts you will use to demonstrate the achievement. You may not have an artifact for each achievement, so you may choose to use a list of brief description instead.

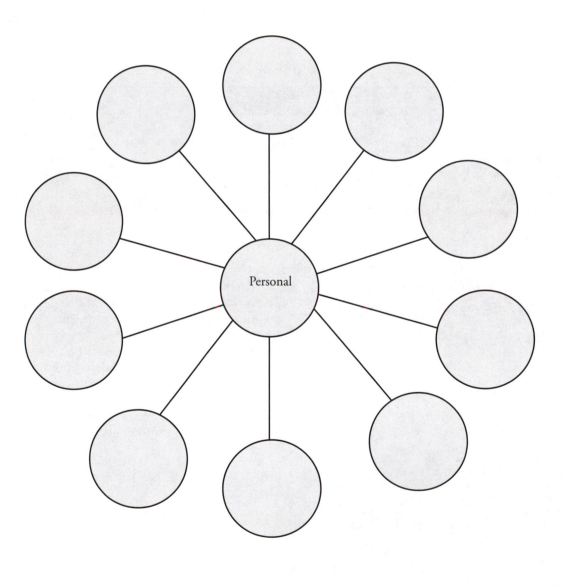

Selecting Guide

Personal: Sample Response

Pictures of me working
with crafts in small
group settings

Pictures of me at state
championship and brief
history of my basketball
experiences

2-page layout of
pictures and
descriptions of
my trips

My love of
crafts

Basketball

Travel

Personal

Self Assessment

Personal

After reviewing your portfolio, grade each of the categories below with a score between 1 and 5 (1 = poor, 3 = good, 5 = excellent). Feel free to make any comments you feel necessary.

Neatness	1 2 3 4 5	Comments:
Organization	1 2 3 4 5	Comments:
Completeness	1 2 3 4 5	Comments:
Content	1 2 3 4 5	Comments:
Relevancy	1 2 3 4 5	Comments:
Flow	1 2 3 4 5	Comments:
Consistency	1 2 3 4 5	Comments:
Visual appearance	1 2 3 4 5	Comments:
Representative of you	1 2 3 4 5	Comments:
Appropriate amount of info	1 2 3 4 5	Comments:

Peer Evaluation

Personal

After reviewing your peer's portfolio, grade each of the categories below with a score between 1 and 5 (1 = poor, 3 = good, 5 = excellent). Feel free to make any comments you feel necessary.

Neatness	1 2 3 4 5	Comments:
Organization	1 2 3 4 5	Comments:
Completeness	1 2 3 4 5	Comments:
Content	1 2 3 4 5	Comments:
Relevancy	1 2 3 4 5	Comments:
Flow	1 2 3 4 5	Comments:
Consistency	1 2 3 4 5	Comments:
Visual appearance	1 2 3 4 5	Comments:
Representative of you	1 2 3 4 5	Comments:
Appropriate amount of info	1 2 3 4 5	Comments:

Peer evaluator's name:

Date:

Sample Portfolio Page

A Short History

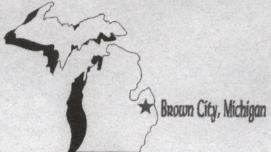

★ Brown City, Michigan

I grew up in Brown City, Michigan, a small town in the state's "thumb region". I graduated from Brown City High School in May, 1995

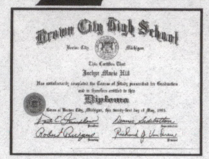

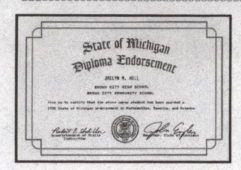

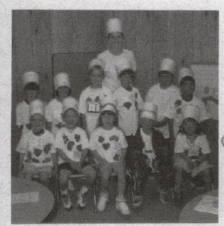

"Celebrate Jesus!"

I was a member of Brown City United Methodist Church and taught Bible School while in High School.

I was also a member of the Girl Scouts of America for 13 years!

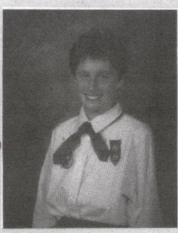

"Honor Guard"

Sample Portfolio Page

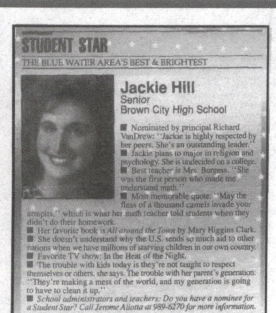

During high school I was named a "Student Star" in the Port Huron Times Herald for my role as Brown City High School's Student Council President.

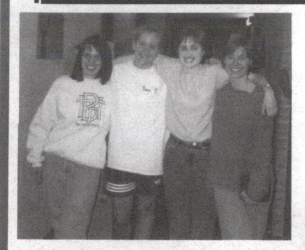

After High School I attended Calvin College in Grand Rapids, Michigan. I attended Calvin for two years.

I am pictured above with my roommates while at Calvin.

At right, I am pictured with a multicultural dance group I took part in called "Gumboots".

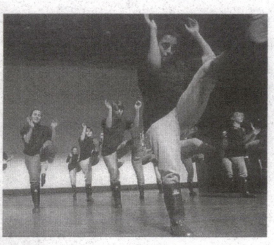

Sample Portfolio Page

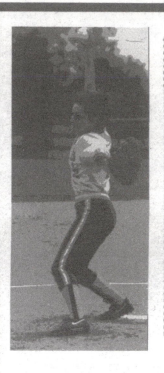

In high school I was a Varsity Athlete in Softball and Basketball.

As a senior, I was captain of the Varsity Softball team.

Hill sisters give Devils a potent 1-2 punch

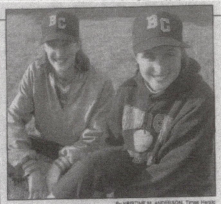

By KRISTINE M. ANDERSON, Times Herald
Karen Hill, left, and her sister Jackie have helped the Brown City softball team get off to an 8-2 start.

While in High School I was a member of the National Honor Society for three years. As a senior I served as an officer of our local chapter.

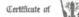

Certificate of Membership

National Honor Society
of
Secondary Schools

This Certifies that
Jaclyn Hill
was selected a member
of the *Brown City High School* Chapter
of the
National Honor Society of Secondary Schools.
Membership is based on
Scholarship, Leadership, Service, and Character.

Given at *Brown City, Michigan*
this   *31st*   day of *March*   *1993*

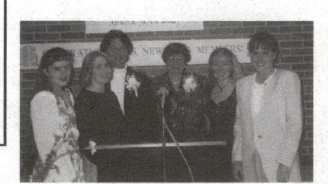

Sample Portfolio Page

SU SaginawValley State University.

(517) 790-4000 • From Midland: (517) 695-5325
7400 Bay Road • University Center, MI 48710

Cheryl E. Easley, Ph.D., R.N.
Dean and Professor
College of Nursing & Allied Health Sciences
(517) 790-4145
Fax: (517) 791-7732
E-mail: ceasley@tardis.svsu.edu

April 28, 1998

Ms. Jaclyn M. Hill
7615 Pine Grove Ln. #1
Saginaw, MI 48604

Dear Ms. Hill:

I am pleased to inform you that you have been selected provisionally to enter the Occupational Therapy Program in the Spring/Summer term of 1998. Full acceptance is pending satisfactory performance on the required courses in which you are currently enrolled. Unless you hear otherwise from my office by Friday, May 8, 1998, your full acceptance has been granted.

Mandatory orientation to the Occupational Therapy Program will occur on Monday, May 11, 1998, at 2:00 p.m. in Ryder West Room 101. Be prepared to register on that day for the following classes

PHE 375	Kinesiology,
PHE 375L	Kinesiology Laboratory, and
OT 302	Foundations in Occupational Therapy.

You will not be assessed a late fee for these classes.

My very best wishes and congratulations as you enter this phase of your education.

Sincerely yours,

Cheryl E. Easley

CEE:reg

I transferred to Saginaw Valley State University in the Fall of 1997.

In the Spring of 1998 I was accepted into the occupational therapy program.

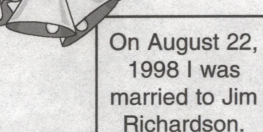

On August 22, 1998 I was married to Jim Richardson.

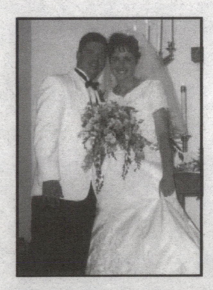

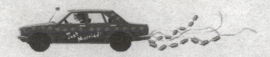

Sample Portfolio Page

PERSONAL INTERESTS

MY FAVORITE ACTIVITIES INCLUDE:

*OUTDOOR ACTIVITIES
   -CAMPING
   -FISHING
   -CANOEING

*COOKING AND BAKING

*GARDENING

*GOLF

*CRAFTING

*MUSIC

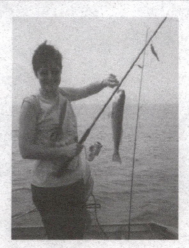

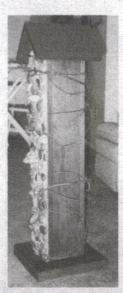

I made this birdhouse with beach stones and wood from old cabinets

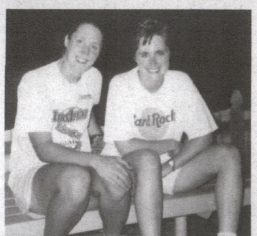

My Sister and I At A "Family Campout"

Create Your Own 15

Case Study

Name: Susan

Age: 53

Current occupation/setting: OTA at a skilled nursing facility

Level of experience: Intermediate

Goal for portfolio: Creating a community outreach program

This is an optional section that you create based on your individual skills, interests, and goals. Perhaps you have done extensive research and you want to demonstrate this area of competence. Maybe occupational therapy is your second career and you want to demonstrate the skills that you developed in your former career and how it relates to your competence as an occupational therapy practitioner. The title and content of this section is up to you—just remember to follow the same basic guidelines for collecting, selecting, organizing, and displaying as you have in the previous sections.

Selecting Guide

Create Your Own

In the circles, write down each achievement, skill, and/or characteristic that you want showcased in your portfolio. Next to the circles, write which artifacts you will use to demonstrate the achievement. You may not have an artifact for each achievement, so you may choose to use a list of brief description instead.

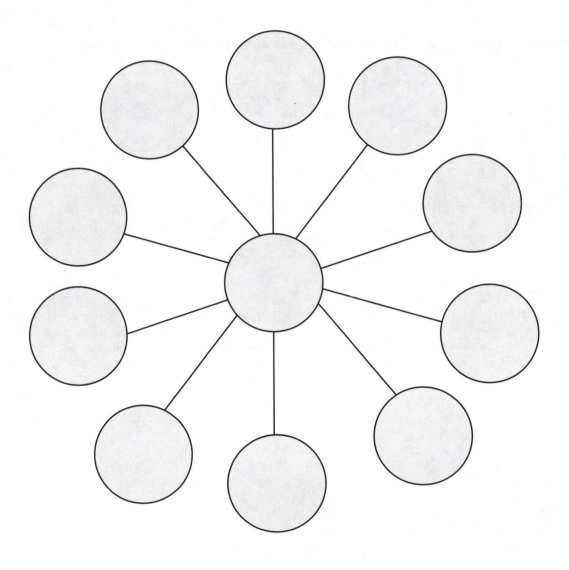

Selecting Guide

Create Your Own: Sample Response

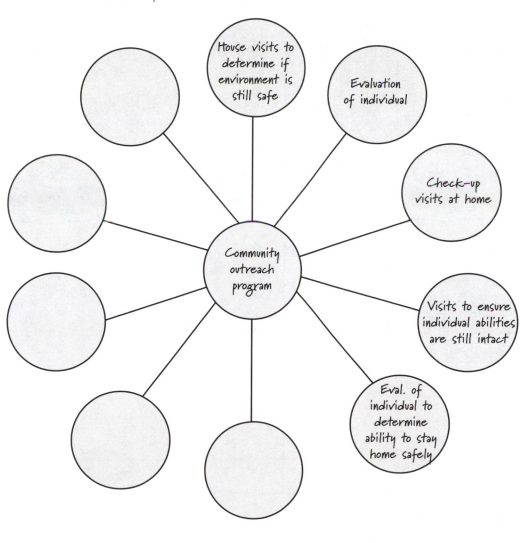

For each service listed below I will use pictures of the evaluations being done, testimonials from clients and their families, and a copy of the evaluation forms that we use.

House visits to determine if environment is still safe

Evaluation of individual

Check-up visits at home

Community outreach program

Visits to ensure individual abilities are still intact

Eval. of individual to determine ability to stay home safely

Self Assessment

Create Your Own

After reviewing your portfolio, grade each of the categories below with a score between 1 and 5 (1 = poor, 3 = good, 5 = excellent). Feel free to make any comments you feel necessary.

Neatness	1 2 3 4 5	Comments:
Organization	1 2 3 4 5	Comments:
Completeness	1 2 3 4 5	Comments:
Content	1 2 3 4 5	Comments:
Relevancy	1 2 3 4 5	Comments:
Flow	1 2 3 4 5	Comments:
Consistency	1 2 3 4 5	Comments:
Visual appearance	1 2 3 4 5	Comments:
Representative of you	1 2 3 4 5	Comments:
Appropriate amount of info	1 2 3 4 5	Comments:

Peer Evaluation

Create Your Own

After reviewing your peer's portfolio, grade each of the categories below with a score between 1 and 5 (1 = poor, 3 = good, 5 = excellent). Feel free to make any comments you feel necessary.

Neatness	1 2 3 4 5	Comments:
Organization	1 2 3 4 5	Comments:
Completeness	1 2 3 4 5	Comments:
Content	1 2 3 4 5	Comments:
Relevancy	1 2 3 4 5	Comments:
Flow	1 2 3 4 5	Comments:
Consistency	1 2 3 4 5	Comments:
Visual appearance	1 2 3 4 5	Comments:
Representative of you	1 2 3 4 5	Comments:
Appropriate amount of info	1 2 3 4 5	Comments:

Peer evaluator's name:

Date:

Sample Portfolio Page

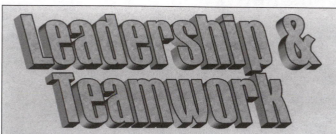

Leadership and Teamwork are abilities that compliment each other and are often interdependent. To be an effective leader, you must understand group dynamics and be able to function as a team member. To be an effective team-member, you must also understand group dynamics and be willing to give of yourself to accomplish the common goal. These attributes are displayed from the very beginning of our lives... in our families, in our school, and in our peer groups. It is from these early learning experiences that we first begin to understand the various roles within a group and how we can function within these various roles. As life progresses our abilities to participate as a team-member and/or a leader improve so that we are more comfortable, effective and productive in these roles.

Leadership Philosophies

Leadership was a main topic in my management class. The following definitions are derived from lectures and discussions in this class. I hold these beliefs and guidelines to be part of my leadership philosophy.

 The role of the leader must be that of a coach— helping the team to prepare and improve, then cheering its successes.

Leadership is the ART of influencing and directing people in such a manner that will win their Respect, Confidence, Obedience, and Loyal Co-operation in achieving a common goal.

Leadership Attributes

Integrity of Character - Moral soundness, honor, trustworthiness, honesty, loyalty, courage (mental/physical)

Sense of Responsibility - See and do what needs to be done, persistence

Professional Competence - Must know the job to keep confidence

Enthusiasm - Ability to find ways to get the job done (usually with a smile)

Emotional Stability - Derived from knowledge, self control, self understanding and knowing your limits

Humanness - Selflessness, concern for others, upholds what is just

— Sample Portfolio Page —

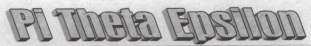

What does Pi Theta Epsilon Mean?

Pi is the first letter of the Greek word for Advancement.

Theta is the first letter in the Greek word for Therapeutic.

Epsilon is the first letter in the Greek word for Occupation.

Therefore, Pi Theta Epsilon means: Advancement in Occupational Therapy

What is Pi Theta Epsilon?

Pi Theta Epsilon is a specialized honor society for occupational therapy students and alumni. This society recognizes and encourages superior scholarship among students enrolled in professional entry-level programs at accredited schools across the United States. The purpose of Pi Theta Epsilon, as stated in the society's Constitution, is:

1. To recognize and encourage scholastic excellence of occupational therapy students;
2. To contribute to the advancement of the field of occupational therapy through the scholarly activities of student and alumni members; and
3. To provide a vehicle for students enrolled in accredited programs in OT to exchange information and to collaborate

What are the requirements?

1. Must be enrolled in an accredited occupational therapy program
2. Is among the top 35% of the class with at least a 3.2 grade point average
3. Fulfills at least two of the following items:
   - Memebrships in professional organizations
   - Prior scholastic recognition and awards
   - Submitted or had papers accepted to local and/or national meetings and publications
   - Documented leadership

I was elected Treasurer of our local chapter. As such I was responsible for all of the financial issues including:

- Collecting dues
- Writing purchase requisition and check requisition forms
- Depositing money collected from all fund-raisers
- Balancing the account in accordance with the university's ledger
- Filling out the forms required by the national office stating who was a member in good standing
- Additionally, I created deposit slips for my use and for future use; created a filing system for past, present and future documents; and organized the balance sheets in a binder.

As a team member I assisted with the following activities:

- Fund-raisers to provide money for charitable organizations and to cover some of the costs for the induction ceremony for new members
- Provided needed supplies for an abused women and children's center
- Collected canned goods for a homeless shelter
- Promoted occupational therapy and Pi Theta Epsilon through bulletin boards, a homecoming banner and several booths at campus events

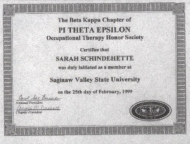

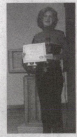

Sample Portfolio Page

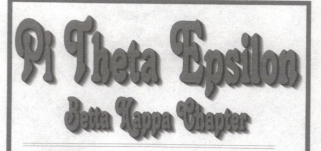

Pi Theta Epsilon
Betta Kappa Chapter

Pi Theta Epsilon is a specialized honor society for Occupational Therapy Students. The organization recognizes exemplary scholarship while promoting service and community participation.

I was inducted into the society on February 25, 1999 at Saginaw Valley State University. I served as an officer during the '99-'00 school year in a public relations position.

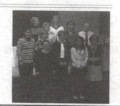

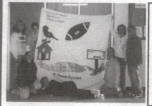

As a member of Pi Theta Epsilon I was involved in many service and campus activities. Our group is pictured at the left with the "Spirit Banner" we made for Homecoming at SVSU. Other activities included a canned food drive, fundraising for a community shelter and participation in SVSU's annual Family Fun Day.

Computer Skills
Programs

I am familiar with a wide variety of programs from personal and professional use including:
Word Processing- Microsoft Word, Word Perfect
Statistical Analysis & Spreadsheets- SSPS, Excel
Home Modification Program- EASE 3.0
Presentations- Powerpoint
Scanner Software- Adobe, Corel, OmniPro
Internet Browsers- Internet Explorer, Netscape

Installing/Set-up

During my employment in the Occupational Therapy department at Saginaw Valley State University I set-up numerous computers and installed a wide variety of programs.

Trouble Shooting

Trouble shooting program errors and training students and faculty in the various programs available were some of my responsibilities while working in the OT department.

Sample Portfolio Page

Organizational Skills

Good organizational skills are exceedingly important throughout my personal and professional life. My definition of organizational skills includes the ability to:

- ✓ visualize the desired outcome
- ✓ determine the steps and resources (including people) necessary to achieve the end result
- ✓ proiritize the steps
- ✓ be flexible and adapt to changing needs and situations to create the best outcome
- ✓ re-evaluate the effectiveness once completed and adjust as needed

These abilities are used during any organizational task, large or small, including: writing papers - organizing a physical space (room, closet, drawer) - organizing your daily routine - organizing a group of people to complete a specific task - etc.

A few examples of what I organized during my employment at Saginaw Valley State University, Occupational Therapy Department:

Student Resource Room - I gathered computers, software, tables and chairs, and reference materials; arranged the furniture to produce the most space; classified, labeled and cross-referenced the reference materials.

Assessment Room - I categorized assessments and developed an efficient system to check out and track the use of assessments.

Lectures and Hand-outs - I created various Powerpoint lectures based on faculty notes, and produced handouts based on lecture material.

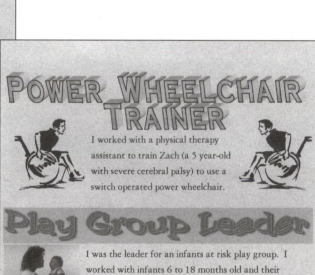

Power Wheelchair Trainer

I worked with a physical therapy assistant to train Zach (a 5 year-old with severe cerebral palsy) to use a switch operated power wheelchair.

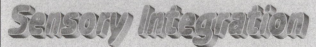

Play Group Leader

I was the leader for an infants at risk play group. I worked with infants 6 to 18 months old and their caregivers. The emphasis was on active play, movement, social interaction and environmental exploration to facilitate development.

Sensory Integration

I initially learned the theories and techniques of sensory integration, including the Wilbarger brushing technique, while participating in interactive workshops. Assessing the need for and implementing sensory integration treatment is a skill that has proven to be indespensible during my fieldwork placement in pediatric rehabilitation, and my jobs in the community mental health and adult rehabilitation settings.

Sample Portfolio Page

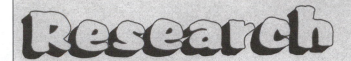

The Use of Physical Agent Modalities (PAM's) in Michigan

Description

A descriptive study on the use of physical agent modalities by occupational therapists practicing in a physical disabilities setting within the state of Michigan.

Procedure

A literature review was completed and a survey constructed to elicit pertinent information from the participants. The survey was sent out to randomly selected occupational therapists practicing in a physical disabilities setting within the state of Michigan. All participants remained anonymous. The survey data was then tallied and entered into a statistical program to analyze the results.

Sample Portfolio Page

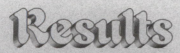

Results

The survey generated a lot of information on several areas of physical agent use including: type of modality used, frequency of use, specific setting in which modalities are used, diagnoses treated with modalities, regulations of use for OT's and PT's, and opinions regarding OT's use of modalities. With the return rate approaching 50 percent we were able to statistically generalize our findings to occupational therapists practicing in a physical disabilities setting within the state of Michigan.

Future of Study

The study generated a high return rate, with an enourmous amount of information regarding a current topic. As a result, the plans for this research include publication and presentation at the national AOTA conference.

Future Research

Date	Topic	Type	Place

A Lifetime of Use

Thinking Critically

Personal Application Guide

What Does Your Portfolio Say?

Self-Evaluation

➤ How your portfolio looks and presents itself says a lot about you. Some qualities do not need direct attention, but are made obvious through indirect means. Examples include neatness, organization, writing skills, and diversity. List three qualities your portfolio indirectly says about you.

➤ How much does your portfolio say? It is important for your portfolio to be complete, but the amount of information on each page should be moderate. Pages should have more than one picture and a heading, but keep in mind that too much narrative is not good either. Look through each page in your portfolio; are there any pages that have too much or too little information on them?

➤ Take a few minutes to look through your completed portfolio and answer the following questions:

How does your portfolio support or promote the field of occupational therapy? How does it answer the question, "What is occupational therapy?"

Personal Application Guide

What Does Your Portfolio Say?

How are your professional goals demonstrated? Is it easy to identify your goals by looking at your portfolio?

Is your portfolio engaging? Is it eye appealing, easy to follow, understand, and read? If yes, explain. If no, what could be changed?

Does your portfolio clearly identify your professional strengths? List three professional strengths and state how each is demonstrated in your portfolio.

List three ways your portfolio could be improved.

Friend and Family Evaluation

Showing your finished portfolio to your closest family members can serve as a valuable critical thinking activity. Choose three people to whom you are close and ask them for honest input regarding your portfolio's strengths and areas that need improvement.

➤   Identify five compliments that these people gave regarding your portfolio.

➤   Identify five areas these people noted for improvement.

Personal Application Guide

Using Your Portfolio to Attain Employment

Imagine taking your portfolio to a job interview and showing the finished product to the potential employer.

➤   Name three interpersonal skills this person may look for:

_____

_____

   How is each demonstrated in your portfolio?

_____

_____

➤   Name three clinical skills this person may look for:

_____

_____

   How is each demonstrated in your portfolio?

_____

_____

➤   Name three good work habits this person may look for:

_____

_____

   How is each demonstrated in your portfolio?

_____

_____

➤   Identify three questions this person may ask you about your profession skills:

_____

_____

   How can you use your portfolio to answer these questions?

_____

_____

➤   Prepare an interview kit including your portfolio, a folder for each person interviewing you (there may be more than one interviewing you at the same time) with a copy of your resume and a list of references inside printed on thick paper, and a notepad and pen so that you can take notes as appropriate.

➤   Practice with a friend. Interview each other until you both feel comfortable with your portfolio layout and how to respond to a potential interview question with a verbal response and reference to your portfolio. This will also build confidence as you remember how much you have accomplished and experienced.

Continuing Development 17

CONTINUITY

The portfolio system and process provide a sense of continuity in the developing and living of our professional and, to an extent, personal lives. The most important benefit may be found not in the completed product, but in the process itself. Discovering who you are, what you believe, what you want, and how you are going to achieve it could be the more intrinsically valuable when you look at the larger picture. Reviewing each of your professional life stages demonstrates the ways in which you may continue to benefit from engaging in the portfolio development process.

PROFESSIONAL DEVELOPMENT

You will develop and continually revise your professional plan, beginning with the decision to become an occupational therapy practitioner. A well maintained portfolio will help to assure that you have the best information available to make decisions regarding formal education and other learning opportunities. It will also record your accomplishments and allow you to review and share your experiences with others. Career advancement and direction changes are based on carefully defined goals and a prescribed plan. Unexpected options and opportunities can also be more easily identified and are weighed within the context of your plan. You may even find that more opportunities are accessible because your plan has prepared you for a wider variety of options.

RECERTIFICATION

Human service providers are being pressed from all sides to clearly define what they do, how they do it, why they should be doing it, and how successful they are at it. Consumers want to receive the most effective care, and reimbursement agents want that care to be provided in an economical manner. Service providers are struggling to remain viable agents and, to do so, must clearly articulate professional philosophy and parameters supported by outcomes research as well as personal professional skills and experience. Occupational therapy is no exception. Toward this end, the National Board for Certification in Occupational Therapy recertification guidelines (www.NBCOT.org) describe a process for planning and pursuing continued professional growth. This includes the development of a professional plan and engaging in a variety of professional development activities. One of the recommended options is the use of a portfolio system to track, support, and showcase professional development. The process NBCOT describes may also be compatible with professional licensing, registration, or certification activity requirements identified by many states. You will need to check with your own local regulatory agencies.

A portfolio can help you track all your accreditation activities with proper organization. When the portfolio system is in place, you will have documentation of all your professional experiences and the related activities right at your fingertips. This is invaluable at all levels of practice, especially when it is time to renew certification. Imagine going into an IRS audit without any of your previous tax returns or receipts! The NBCOT recertification process is new and will likely continue to evolve. The portfolio system provides an organized and fluid means of planning and documenting your participation in the various approved professional activities, whatever your accreditation needs. This is a process that will last throughout your career and is well worth the rather large initial investment of time and more moderate upkeep.

The NBCOT (www.NBCOT.org) currently has 29 approved professional development activities. They are working toward providing guidelines and forms for each of those activities. A portfolio system will help you organize and track the activities in which you choose to engage and highlight the results. The required accompanying information must include the original documentation or a copy of all related professional development activities for one year following your certification renewal. Many of these activities are ongoing and can be recorded in chart form to more easily track participation. Suggestions for detailing and verifying your progress are based in NBCOT (www.NBCOT.org) recommendations for recertification but will be helpful for your own personal use as well. A list of suggested topics is provided regarding the type of information you will need to keep. Each topic will require individualized data collection and organization. A sample chart is provided for each of the following activity types, which may be adapted to meet your individual needs.

✳ Receiving specialty certifications

1. Dates and time spent

2. Course provider and presenter(s)

3. Course objectives, content, learning activities

4. Certification earned

5. Continuing activities required

✳ Engaging in a mentoring relationship

Several recordkeeping activities are required to track this relationship whether you are the mentor or the mentee (NBCOT***)

1. Goals of the mentee

2. The mentor's plan of instruction

3. Dates and times mentoring occurs

4. Evaluation procedures wherein the mentee evaluates the mentor and the mentor evaluates the mentee

5. A mutual review of the feedback by each member and documented improvement

✳ Independent learning activities

Reading approved materials and writing an analysis

1. Annotated bibliography of materials selected and inclusive dates of study

2. Written analysis of each selection demonstrating how the content applies to your practice area and impacts your clientele

✳ Formal academic coursework, audited academic courses, online courses, and external self-study opportunities may all be verified through transcripts and certificates of completion. You may also want to write a short analysis of how the individual course or set of courses applies to your current position or professional development plan. A list of accomplishments could provide a summary of activities but would not stand alone as proof of accomplishment

✳ Occupational therapy related publications may be tracked through the use of an annotated bibliography of your works

✳ Professional study groups should maintain records evidencing the following features

1. Three to 20 participants

2. The group should meet at least three times for a minimum of one hour per session

3. Document learning goals

4. Document the learning plan to meet the stated goals

5. Minutes should be kept for each meeting

6. When the goals have been met an analysis should be written summarizing what was learned, how it applied to each member's role, and implications for further learning

✳ Other

The remaining professional development activities embody extensive research and content. You will want to keep the original work separately, and safely, in your file cabinet. An abstract of the activity including dates of involvement and outcomes can be placed in your portfolio

1. Scholarly research and outcomes studies

2. Development of instructional materials using alternative media

3. Program development is not included in NBCOT guidelines but certainly has a place in professional development and the application of knowledge and skills

Professional Presentations

Making Presentations on Occupational Therapy Related Topics

Date(s)	Topic	Location	Audience	PDU value

Professional Development Activities

Attending Workshops, Seminars, Lectures, and Conferences

Date(s)	Type (lecture, seminar, etc.)	Topic	Location, presenter(s)	PDU value

Continuing Education Activities

Attending Employer-Provided Continuing Education Activities

Date(s)	Topic	Location	Presenter(s)	PDU value

Teaching Experiences

Guest Teaching in an Academic Course

Date(s)	Course, credit(s)	Location	Content	PDU value

Community Service/Volunteer

Services That Advance Occupational Therapy Skills and Experiences

Date(s)	Name of organization	Description of activities	Outcomes	PDU value

Fieldwork Supervision

Level II Fieldwork Direct Primary Supervision

Date(s)	Name of student	Location, setting	Level I or II	PDU value

Professional Manuscript Reviews

Reviewing Professional Manuscripts and Proposals

Date(s)	Title	Pages, content	Publisher	PDU value

Self-Study Activities

Independent Learning and Study Activities

Date(s)	Type (journal, study groups, etc.)	Topic	Outcome, application	PDU value

Bibliography

Abbott, A. (1988). *Professional choices: Values at work.* National Association of Social Workers, Inc., USA.

American Occupational Therapy Association, (1994). Occupational therapy code of ethics. *American Journal of Occupational Therapy, 48,* 1037-1038.

American Occupational Therapy Association. (1994). Uniform terminology for occupational therapy (3rd ed.). *American Journal of Occupational Therapy, 48,* 1047-1054.

American Occupational Therapy Association. (2002). *Occupational therapy framework: Domain and process.* Retrieved 2004 from http:// www.aota.org/members /area2/docs/frame.pdf.

American Occupational Therapy Association. (1972). OT: Its definition and function. *American Journal of Occupational Therapy, 26,* 204.

Bateman, T. & Snell, S. (2004). *Management: The new competitive landscape.* Boston: McGraw-Hill Irwin.

Bureau of Labor Statistics, U.S. Department of Labor. Occupational therapist assistants and aides. *Occupational Outlook Handbook.* (2002-03 ed.). Retrieved December 2, 2004 from http://bls.gov/oco/ocos166.htm.

Dunn, W., & Campbell., P.H. (1991). Designing pediatric occupational therapeutic service provision. In W. Dunn (Ed.), *Pediatric occupational therapy: Facilitating effective service provision.* (pp. 139-160). Thorofare, NJ: SLACK Incorporated.

Kanny, E. (1993). Core values and attitudes of occupational therapy practice. *American Journal of Occupational Therapy, 47,* 1085-1086.

Meyer, A. (1922). Philosophy of occupation therapy. *Archives of Occupational Therapy, 1,* 1-10. (Reprinted in *American Journal of Occupational Therapy, 31,* 639-642, 1977).

National Board for Certification in Occupational Therapy Web site. March 1, 2004. from http://www.nbcot.org.

Punwar, A. (1994). *Occupational therapy principles and practice.* Baltimore: Williams & Wilkins.

Sabonis-Chafee, B., & Hussey, S. M. (1998). *Introduction to occupational therapy.* (2nd ed). Philadelphia: Mosby.

Sullivan, W. M. (1995). *Work and integrity: The crisis and promise of professionalism in America.* New York: Harper Collins Publishers, Inc.

Webster's new world dictionary. (1990). Cleveland, OH: Warner Books.

Index